THE DIABETES SELF-CARE METHOD

The
Diabetes
Self-Care Method

Third Edition

Charles M. Peterson, M.D.
and Lois Jovanovic, M.D.

THE BREAKTHROUGH PROGRAM OF
SELF-MANAGEMENT THAT WILL HELP
YOU LEAD A HEALTHIER LIFE

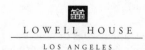

LOWELL HOUSE

LOS ANGELES

NTC/Contemporary Publishing Group

Library of Congress Cataloging-in-Publication Data

Peterson, C.M.
 .The diabetes self-care method : the breakthrough program of self-management that will help you lead a better, freer, more normal life/Charles M. Peterson.
p. cm.
Includes index.
ISBN 0-929923-29-4
ISBN 0-7373-0017-5
1. Diabetes. 2. Self-care, Health.
II. Title.
RC660.P42   1990
616.4'62—dc20   90-2142
                                                             CIP

Published by Lowell House, a division of NTC/Contemporary Publishing Group, Inc., 4255 West Touhy Avenue, Lincolnwood, Illinois 60646-1975 U.S.A.   .

Design by Robert S. Tinnon

Printed and bound in the United States of America
International Standard Book Number: 0-7373-0017-5
10 9 8 7 6 5 4 3 2 1

To Caroline Elizabeth and Karen

Contents

Introduction

It is hard to believe that this book is now over twenty years old in its several editions. It was first written at a time before the term empowerment became so popular but that, in fact, was the original aim of the book. The belief behind the book has always been that with the proper tools and skills, persons with diabetes can take charge and manage the condition in a way that allows near normal blood sugars to be attained over time. With this management, the long term problems of diabetes can be avoided.

The book continues to stem from research conducted in recent years on diabetes and its secondary complications. The main object of this research has been to find out what causes the complications of diabetes and whether these problems can be prevented or corrected. Through research, we have found that many complications can be prevented. Even more encouraging, we learned that some complications may even be reversed through a good program of diabetes management.

It is clear not only that diabetic persons can manage their own disease but that many do it exceptionally well. Our studies show that the main problem for persons with diabetes is how best to achieve and maintain such management. The health professional can teach the principles and practices of good management, but it is up to the diabetic individual to maintain his or her own program.

This book summarizes our approach to optimum control of diabetes and offers a practical approach, employed successfully by persons with diabetes, to good self-management. It explains why control is necessary and presents the "tricks" and systems used to achieve "control" or how to "Take Charge of Your Diabetes," as this book was originally titled. This third version also includes completely revised information on the many new drugs now available, as well as information on the new "designer insulins."

Patients often ask what they should not do or what they should avoid. The answer is simple. There is nothing they need avoid or should not do because they have diabetes. Persons with diabetes do have to be a "bit smarter" to have these degrees of freedom as well as work a little harder but the extra dedication invariably brings the desired results. In fact, diabetic persons often have an advantage over other people as a result of their increased knowledge of health maintenance. It is our hope that the information in this book about nutrition, exercise, and better living habits will benefit not only persons with diabetes but also their families and friends.

1

Diabetes and Its Complications

What is diabetes? The disease called *diabetes mellitus* has been known to humankind for thousands of years. Egyptian scribes alluded to the disease and its classical symptoms in the famed Ebers Papyrus around 1500 B.C.

Early physicians gave the disease its name from a Greek word meaning "siphon" or "to run through," after observing that persons afflicted with this condition passed excessive quantities of urine. These early medical observers also noted a sickly sweet odor in the urine of persons with diabetes. This observation led to the development of a rather primitive diagnostic test that required tasting the urine to determine the extent of its sweetness. It also led to a second word to complete the description of the disease, *mellitus*, from the Latin for "honey." Thus, the name *diabetes mellitus* tells us that the disease involves a passage of a sweet substance through the body.

It was not until two hundred years ago that this sweet substance was identified as glucose (sugar). The question then remained: where did this glucose come from and why did it accumulate in the urine of persons with diabetes?

Today we know that this accumulation results from a buildup of glucose in the blood, or hyperglycemia. When the body cannot use or store glucose properly, unused amounts remain in the bloodstream. Eventually this level exceeds a point which the body accepts as normal, and spills over into the urine.

Although laboratory methods for measuring blood and urine glucose were developed in the nineteenth century, little could be done for persons with diabetes until 1921, when Frederick Banting and Charles Best of Canada isolated the body's glucose-regulating hormone, insulin. Their discovery dramatically changed the concept of diabetes treatment, which had been limited to near-starvation diets in an attempt to decrease the body's need for insulin. With insulin injections, persons with diabetes could eat more normally and gain sufficient control of the disease to live a more productive life.

HOW DOES INSULIN WORK?

Although insulin has improved countless numbers of lives, it is not a cure for diabetes. Insulin only helps to regulate the body's blood glucose levels. How does the regulatory system work? In a normally functioning body, blood glucose levels are regulated by what is described as a "closed-loop system" (see Figure 1.1). The nondiabetic person has a constant glucose sensor in the pancreas which responds to an elevation in blood glucose by putting out a little insulin to lower the glucose level. In persons with diabetes, however, the loop is not completed because the pancreas either can no longer produce insulin or produces it in insufficient amounts to bring down the blood glucose. The result is too much glucose circulating in the bloodstream. The broken loop must be mended with another source of insulin, injected by the diabetic himself. Alternatively, some people with diabetes

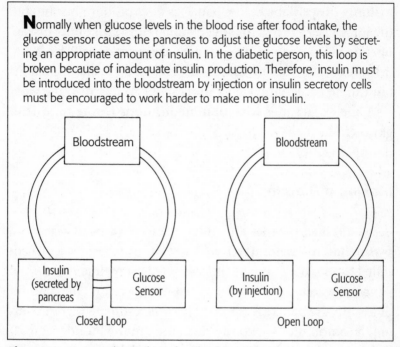

Normally when glucose levels in the blood rise after food intake, the glucose sensor causes the pancreas to adjust the glucose levels by secreting an appropriate amount of insulin. In the diabetic person, this loop is broken because of inadequate insulin production. Therefore, insulin must be introduced into the bloodstream by injection or insulin secretory cells must be encouraged to work harder to make more insulin.

Figure 1.1 How Insulin Works in the Bloodstream

can use medicines to help them make more insulin or make them more sensitive to the insulin they do make. These oral drugs that increase insulin production or sensitivity are discussed in Chapter 3.

TYPES OF DIABETES

Not all diabetic patients have to inject insulin. Diabetes generally appears in two forms, known as type 1 and type 2. The type 1 individual's pancreas cannot produce insulin. Therefore, the person with type 1 diabetes needs insulin from another source: either injected, transplanted, or through genetic engineering of other cells to make insulin. In type 2 diabetes, also known as maturity-onset diabetes, the pancreas does produce insulin, but the body resists the circulating insulin. This form of the disease often tends to occur in persons who are overweight. Type 2 diabetic persons are not necessarily dependent on insulin injections but can be treated through a program of proper diet and exercise, and sometimes with oral medications (more on this in Chapter 3).

Making a Diagnosis

Because it is sometimes difficult to tell which type of diabetes a person has, it is helpful to have a test which measures a protein called C-peptide. This protein is secreted every time the normal pancreas secretes a molecule of insulin. Therefore, the amount of insulin the pancreas is making can be estimated by measuring the amount of C-peptide circulating in the bloodstream. If little or no C-peptide is present, we know that the person has type 1 diabetes—that is, the person's pancreas is not helping to control glucose levels in the blood. C-peptide is produced only by the body, so even if a person injected insulin before the test, the contribution of the pancreas could still be judged.

Insulin itself is often taken up by the liver, so measuring insulin in the blood after it has gone through the liver is not as reliable a test of pancreatic function as measuring C-peptide. Therefore, to find out whether your pancreas is working for you and to what extent, your physician can measure your C-peptide levels, either fasting or after a meal, when your blood glucose is elevated, so the pancreas will be challenged to give its "best effort."

C-peptide also provides an indication of whether you may eventually need to take insulin or not. For example, if you are overweight and have relatively high C-peptide levels, you may not need to take extra insulin but may do fine just by losing weight and exercising. However, if your C-peptide levels are low, your physician may want you to begin insulin injections relatively soon because your insulin output is not able to keep up with your insulin needs. This is especially true in type 2 diabetic persons who have a high degree of "insulin resistance." A falling C-peptide level may be indicative of the pancreas reaching a state of exhaustion in these cases, and therefore, the need for insulin may be relatively urgent.

SECONDARY COMPLICATIONS OF DIABETES

Although diabetes is defined by having a high blood glucose level, the situation becomes more complicated because of all the harmful problems that can result over the short and long term from hyperglycemia. These resultant problems are referred to as the "sequelae," or secondary, complications of diabetes.

Acidosis

Another problem for persons with diabetes, in addition to hyperglycemia, is a condition called acidosis. Acidosis results when the body cannot properly break down the glucose that fuels cells. The body begins to burn its own fat and muscle for energy, and the acid waste products accumulate in the blood.

The little bit of insulin that is present in the type 2 diabetic person is generally enough to prevent the occurrence of fat breakdown and acidosis. Nevertheless, if the body is subject to infection or serious stress, acidosis may occur in type 2 patients as well.

Glucose and acid accumulations in the blood are warning signs of potentially disastrous problems. At first, the diabetic person may feel weak or giddy and a little sick to the stomach. If left unchecked, these warning signs may result in loss of consciousness and the need for emergency hospitalization. Generally, these severe problems can be avoided with even the most modest approach to diabetes management.

Hypoglycemia

Hypoglycemia is the most common complication of diabetes, especially in persons taking insulin, but it can also occur in persons with type 2 diabetes on oral medication. Therefore, it is critical for every person with diabetes as well as friends and family to be aware of the feelings and signs associated with low blood glucose levels. Low blood sugars can be deadly not only because the body needs fuel from sugar but especially because the brain is the most sensitive organ to low blood glucose levels and muscles do not work well with a poor glucose supply. It is impossible to perform mental and physical tasks such as driving a car to the best of your ability when your blood sugar is low. In fact, in the state of California, if you have diabetes and are found to be driving erratically with a blood glucose of less than 90 mg/dl, you will lose your license. Every person with diabetes should be aware of blood glucose levels before and while driving an automobile. Chapter 10 deals with this problem of low blood sugars in some detail.

Vascular Disease

Diabetic persons may avoid the problems of hyperglycemia and acidosis and still be vulnerable to other secondary problems of diabetes. Persons with diabetes and even persons without diabetes but with increasingly poor glucose tolerance have an increased risk of vascular disease including heart attacks, stroke, and impaired circulation, particularly in the hands and feet as well as eye and kidney disease discussed below. Since diabetic patients may have other risk factors associated with these problems—obesity, sedentary lifestyle, high blood lipids, cigarette smoking—it is difficult to determine which factor is primary in leading to the high incidence of vascular disease in a given individual with diabetes. However, there is now a general agreement that glucose elevations over time increase the risk of both forms of vascular disease. Yet many of these risk factors can be reduced.

Neuropathy

Another secondary complication in diabetes is neuropathy, a condition affecting the nerves and marked by a loss of sensation, especially in the limbs. The diabetic person may feel a burning, tingling, or "funny" sensation in the hands or feet along any network of involved nerves. He or she may also feel slightly weak because the nerves are not conducting messages correctly to the muscles. Poor conduction of messages by nerves may lead to sexual dysfunction and impotence if the nerves involved with erection or other sexual functions are affected. These changes can be avoided with good glucose control. In fact, some nerve changes can actually be reversed when returning to more normal glucose levels over periods of months to years.

Vision Problems

Diabetes may lead to several types of eye afflictions. The most common is retinopathy, which seems to worsen with the duration of the diabetes. In diabetic retinopathy, the fragile blood

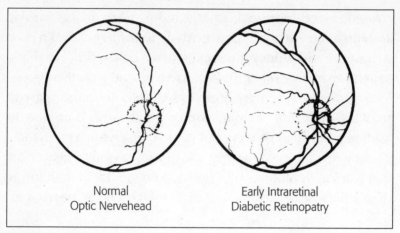

Normal
Optic Nervehead

Early Intraretinal
Diabetic Retinopatry

Figure 1.2 Retina with and without Retinopathy

vessels that nourish the back lining of the eye (retina) weaken and balloon (see Figure 1.2). Eventually, the vessel walls may burst, and severe bleeding will occur, blocking light to the retina and resulting in cloudy vision. Photocoagulation (laser therapy) has been used to slow or halt the progression of this eye complication, but the best therapy is still prevention. Experiments in animals and humans have consistently shown that retinopathy can be prevented by good control of blood glucose levels. Further good news comes from France, where research studies have shown that retinopathy may actually be reversed with optimum control of the diabetes if the condition is identified early in the course of eye disease and good control is maintained throughout the years. Even if eye disease has progressed to a point where there is danger of losing eyesight, then excellent therapies are available to preserve vision with the use of laser treatments to the eye.

In addition to retinal changes, persons with diabetes seem to be susceptible to cataract formation. Why this is so is not thoroughly understood. One explanation is that the proteins or structural molecules which form the lens of the eye tend to react to abnormal amounts of blood glucose. If diabetes is not under control, excess glucose will attach to the lens proteins and alter their composition and shape. When this happens, the protein forms opaque areas in the lens. This is known as a cataract. It follows then that the lower the blood glucose, the less likely the lens is to form a cataract. Chapter 2 discusses eye problems associated with diabetes in further detail.

Kidney Problems

Diabetes also takes its toll on the body's major filtering system—the kidneys. Through an ingenious system, the kidneys remove waste materials from the bloodstream where they have been deposited by the cells. This filtration of waste is carried on by the glomerulus, a sievelike structure, which then passes the filtered materials into the tubules of the kidneys, which in turn reabsorb what the body can reuse.

Even when operating at peak efficiency, the kidneys can reabsorb only so much glucose and water. If too much glucose is present, it remains in the tubules and is passed out with urine and the sugar takes more water along with it. This excess water and sugar is called *polyuria*. Along with excess thirst, *polydipsia*, and excess hunger and food consumption, *polyphagia*, these three "polys" are what the ancients used to characterize persons with diabetes. Urinary tract infection is more likely to occur in diabetic patients, partly because high urinary glucose levels encourage bacterial growth. High blood glucose also may cause the kidneys to undergo destructive changes and eventually cease to function. Usually, the glomerulus becomes damaged with an expansion of mesangium which may destroy the entire structure of the filtering system.

Here again, research studies offer new hope for persons with diabetes. The University of Minnesota Kidney Transplant Unit has done considerable work in this area, with promising results. Their investigations show that normal kidneys transplanted in persons with uncontrolled diabetes tend to develop diabetic kidney changes within a period of four years. In another study, a kidney with damage to the glomerulus due to diabetes was transplanted in a nondiabetic rat, and the changes were reversed to normal. Again, it seems that there is something in the internal environment of diabetes which predisposes them to these kidney changes. If this environment—high circulating blood glucose—is brought under control, the damaging changes may be reversed. A number of human studies has proven that good glucose control can prevent kidney changes. The most well known and largest of these studies is known as the Diabetes and Control Complications Trial (DCCT). The DCCT was a large, randomized (people were assigned treatment groups by chance like a lottery), prospective (it watched people over many years) trial in persons with type 1 diabetes with high statistical power. It ended years of debate by conclusively showing the following:

1. Good control of glucose for more than two to three years prevents diabetes-related diseases of the eye, kidney, and nerves.
2. Good control of glucose helps save the pancreas from losing its ability to make insulin. The more insulin the pancreas can make, the easier it is to control glucose levels over time. Therefore, the argument that persons with diabetes should maintain as near-normal glucose levels as possible becomes stronger with each passing year.

Other Effects on Blood Chemistry

In addition to glucose levels, other aspects of blood chemistry are affected by diabetes. Diabetic patients are prone to have high levels of blood lipids such as cholesterol and triglycerides. Some cholesterol-containing molecules appear to be more harmful than others. These are the low-density lipoproteins (LDL) and very low-density lipoproteins (VLDL), which form deposits in cells and vessels. These deposits lead to premature hardening of the arteries.

On the other side, high-density lipoproteins (HDL) help the body to eliminate harmful cholesterol from the cells. In poorly controlled diabetes, the ratio of this protective lipoprotein to the harmful type is quite low, and levels of triglycerides and cholesterol are high. As the diabetes is brought under control, the situation is reversed. Triglyceride and cholesterol levels decrease, and the ratio of the beneficial high-density lipoprotein to the damaging low-density type increases.

High circulating blood glucose also interferes with the white blood cells—the body's defense against bacterial invaders. Because of this, diabetic persons are more susceptible to infections of all types when the disease is out of control. Once the blood glucose levels are lowered toward normal, the white cells again begin to function normally in their safeguarding role.

The red blood cells, too, are influenced by high circulating glucose. The red cell contains hemoglobin, the substance that carries oxygen from the lungs to the tissues. In poorly controlled diabetes, these red cells have been found to age more rapidly than otherwise. They are also subject to changes in the hemoglobin, a protein with a specific composition. In the diabetic environment, circulating glucose will attach to the hemoglobin and alter its structure. When this happens, the altered hemoglobin cannot release its oxygen as readily to the tissues.

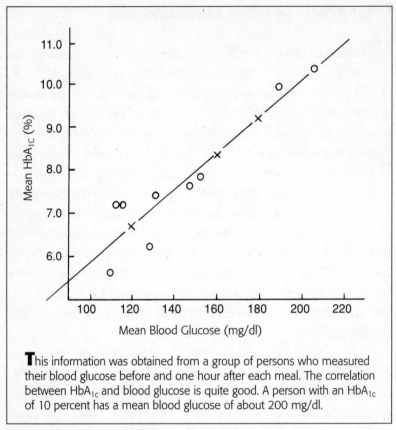

This information was obtained from a group of persons who measured their blood glucose before and one hour after each meal. The correlation between HbA$_{1c}$ and blood glucose is quite good. A person with an HbA$_{1c}$ of 10 percent has a mean blood glucose of about 200 mg/dl.

Figure 1.3 A Comparison of HbA$_{1c}$ with Mean Blood Glucose

Measurement of the amount of this glucose-hemoglobin combination—called glycated hemoglobin, glycosylated hemoglobin, or hemoglobin A$_{1c}$ (HbA$_{1c}$)—in the blood is a useful tool to monitor diabetes control. The approximate life span of the red cell is 120 days. As it gets older, the cell accumulates more glucose-hemoglobin combination, especially if it is circulating in a high glucose environment. Thus the higher the blood glucose and the longer it has been elevated, the greater the level of hemoglobin A$_{1c}$ in the blood (see Figure 1.3). By measuring the amount of hemoglobin A_{1c}, the average blood glucose can be determined over the past several weeks to months. This provides a more accurate assessment of diabetes control than blood glucose measurements, which can fluctuate wildly over short periods of time.

There are a number of proteins that are modified by glucose in a manner similar to the way hemoglobin is modified (glycosylated). Measurement of all of these modified hemoglobins in the red blood cells also give an average of the blood glucose level over the past six to eight weeks.

Another major blood component—platelets—is apt to lose its effectiveness in uncontrolled diabetes. Platelets rush to plug the leaks that result when you cut or wound yourself. In persons with high blood glucose levels, these platelets tend to clot more readily. As the blood glucose level decreases, the platelets once again return to normal and are no longer hypercoagulable.

One of the other components of the body's clotting system, fibrinogen, is used in excessive amounts by poorly controlled diabetic persons. In fact, the rate of utilization appears to be about twice that of nondiabetic people. Again, when the diabetic is brought under control, the fibrinogen life span returns to normal, and the person with diabetes with normal blood glucose is not as vulnerable to form a clot. If clots occur in the brain, a stroke may occur. If clots occur in the vessels of the heart, the person may suffer a heart attack or myocardial infarct.

Effects on Growth in Children

Poor control of blood glucose levels has been found to stunt the growth and development of children with diabetes. Although the administration of insulin can save their lives, poorly controlled diabetic children do not seem to develop and grow as well as their nondiabetic peers. If relatively normal blood

Table 1.1 Outlook for Complications of Diabetes

Problem	Preventable?	Reversible?	Time to Reversal
Elevated glycosylated hemoglobin	yes	yes	12 weeks
Elevated triglycerides	yes	yes	3 weeks
Elevated cholesterol	yes	yes	6–10 weeks
Poor white-cell function and vulnerability to infection	yes	yes	3 weeks
Neuropathy			
Early	yes	yes	50% improvement in 9 months
Late	yes	not known	
Retinopathy			
Early	yes	probably	
Late	yes	doubtful	
Capillary basement membrane thickening	yes	yes	9 months
Poor outcome of pregnancy	yes		
Vulnerability to clotting			
platelet function	yes	yes	1 week
Fibrinogen turnover	yes	yes	hours
Large-vessel disease of legs	yes		
Early	yes	yes	9 months*
Late	yes	not known	

*With exercise and nonsmoking

glucose levels are maintained in these children, they can progress physically at a normal rate and even "catch up" if good glucose control is initiated in time.

Problems During Pregnancy

Pregnant diabetic women present a special set of problems. Loss of the baby during pregnancy occurs much more frequently in diabetic than in nondiabetic mothers-to-be. In addition, there are apt to be more problems at the time of delivery, and there is an increased possibility of abnormalities in the infant if the diabetes is not well controlled throughout pregnancy. Optimum control of diabetes before and during pregnancy can improve the chances of having a normal baby to the same degree as the nondiabetic mother (see Chapter 8).

And so the case for good diabetes management continues to mount with increasing evidence that certain secondary complications cannot only be prevented, but even be reversed. A current research effort is concerned with identifying which problems are reversible and at what point this can be done. Table 1.1 summarizes some of the problems associated with diabetes and indicates whether they can be prevented or reversed, based on the information we have available today.

2

Measuring Your Health Status

One of the best ways to learn about diabetes is to talk to someone who has the disease and manages it well. We have found it extremely helpful to use our own patients' experiences to explain some of the problems other persons with diabetes face. (In such instances, we have changed the names and actual situations.)

Rita, now thirty, has had diabetes for almost as long as she could remember. She never exercised, and ignored habits of good control so that she was always spilling about 1 or 2 percent glucose in her urine. Her skin was pasty, and little bumps had formed around her eyes over the past few years, an indication that her blood lipids were high. Rita's pituitary gland had been removed many years ago when she contracted severe eye disease. (The pituitary, the master control for many other hormone-producing glands, rests at the base of the brain below the optic nerves.)

Because of her eye problems and numerous low blood glucose (hypoglycemic) reactions, Rita was afraid to try to control her diabetes.

Rita was hospitalized so that she could be taught the step-by-step procedures to achieve and maintain good control. After her diabetes was brought under control, Rita's blood lipid levels dropped tremendously. The triglycerides dropped almost immediately, and blood cholesterol levels decreased about six weeks after control was established. Hemoglobin A_{1c} levels also came down three to four weeks after the diabetes was brought under control and continued to drop over the next three months (see Figure 2.1). Rita's skin lost its pasty color, and the lipid marks around her eyes disappeared completely. Since she was not plummeting from such heights of hyperglycemia, her symptoms of hypoglycemia also improved. She then had to train herself to find new clues to her low sugars so she could maintain better control without the fear of disastrous lows.

In Rita's case, hospitalization was necessary to correct long-neglected problems and to train her to recognize her own symptoms and signs of low blood sugars. If you are already well into good self-management skills, however, you can now take three extra measures toward maintaining optimum control of your diabetes:

1. Periodically evaluate the status of potential long-term complications, paying particular attention to your eyes, kidneys, and blood lipids.
2. Know how well you are managing your diabetes over a set time period.
3. Employ some means to measure your own blood glucose levels so that you can respond to any changes appropriately with diet, exercise, or medication. You may

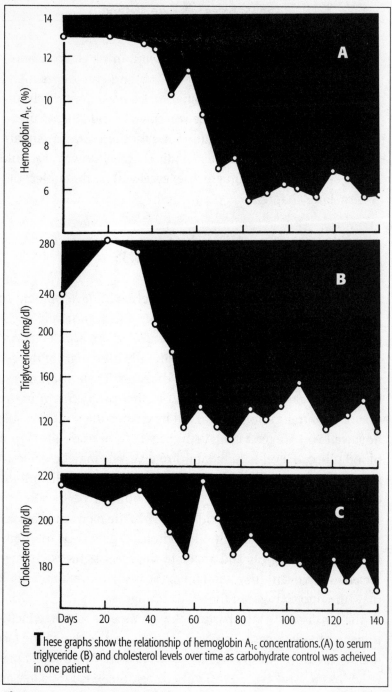

These graphs show the relationship of hemoglobin A₁c concentrations.(A) to serum triglyceride (B) and cholesterol levels over time as carbohydrate control was acheived in one patient.

Figure 2.1 Measuring Hemoglobin A₁c

be doing this now by testing your urine glucose, but this is not nearly as helpful as blood glucose testing. Fortunately, present technologies make it fairly simple for you to learn to take your own blood glucose measurement. The optimum time for these measurements will be discussed later in this chapter. How you should respond to blood glucose levels will be the subject of later chapters.

EYE EXAMINATIONS

How do you evaluate your status in terms of development of complications of diabetes? You probably visit your family physician at least once a year, but do you also see an eye doctor annually? If you don't, you should. Virtually every part of the eye can be adversely affected by your diabetes. Then, too, the eye serves as an early-warning system of other problems. Your eye doctor (ophthalmologist) can tell by examining your eyes just how well you are managing your diabetes. For example, if your blood glucose level is high, abnormal vessels may be detected in the conjunctiva, the outer membrane of the eyeball, and the cornea, or lens covering, may become wrinkled.

Your eye doctor will also look at the iris, the pigmented area of your eye, which may develop little holes if glucose is too high. New vessels will grow and attach to the eye, or glucose storage material (glycogen) may build up in the iris. The eye muscle itself may undergo changes in the vessel linings.

The lens is one of the parts of the eye most sensitive to elevations in blood glucose. This sensitivity, in part, is due to the fact that we are born with most of the lens protein or structural material that we will ever have. Furthermore, the lens grows like an onion, from the outside inward. Therefore, whatever damage a lens protein undergoes will generally be there for the rest of our lives.

If sugar reacts with lens tissue, it becomes more vulnerable to forming an area that cannot transmit light, an area called a cataract. The reaction with sugar leads to clumping together of the lens proteins, and a cataract can develop. This process can happen to nondiabetic individuals over their lifetime. Such a process is referred to as a cataract of aging, or brown cataract, because of its color. Persons with diabetes are more vulnerable to this process because the level of blood glucose is more apt to be high. The way to prevent early cataract formation from glucose or sugar reacting with the lens is obviously to keep blood sugar as near normal as possible.

It is also important to have your lens examined with the rest of the eye and to remind your eye doctor and general physician that you have diabetes. Some medicines may also promote cataract formation—for example, allopurinol, a medicine for gout taken by many persons with diabetes. Another way of protecting yourself from early cataracts is to protect the eye from ultraviolet (UV) light exposure, which also may induce cataracts. Wear sunglasses that screen out ultraviolet light whenever you're outdoors, especially in bright sunlight or when in the snow or over water. If you wear regular glasses, ask for the kind with a UV filter as well. They will not be dark glasses but will screen out the harmful UV light.

Above all, your eye doctor will be concerned about your retina (which receives light and transmits images to the brain). Any interference with the structure of the retina will obscure vision. Your eye doctor may inject a fluorescent dye into your vein to study the retinal vessels or perhaps use one of the newer methods to evaluate the smaller vessels. The number of protective cells around these vessels has been noted to decrease in persons with diabetes, and the vessels appear to have less blood circulating in them than in the nondiabetic person's eye. Thus some areas of the eye may not get as much oxygen as others. Small "balloons" may develop and increase in size as diabetes continues out of control. These balloons (aneurysms) may break, and severe bleeding can occur within or above the retina. Excess fluid (exudates) may accumulate in parts of the retina—a warning sign of vascular problems in the eye. All of these factors may cause the retina to detach from its anchor at the back of the eye and impair vision.

Between the retina in the back of the eye and the lens in the front is a ball of clear gelatin-type material called the vitreous humor. The vitreous itself may become totally clouded if severe bleeding occurs. In addition, it may retract away from the retina and lead to visual impairment. The optic nerve which carries all the pooled nerves attached to the retina in one large bundle to the brain is apt to degenerate in poorly controlled diabetic persons.

Diabetes is not the only cause of these eye problems, but persons with diabetes are more prone to significant vision changes and should be especially careful to check the fit of their glasses. Focal length may change from time to time in anyone, but especially in persons with diabetes. Your eye doctor will help to recognize significant vision changes early.

CHECKING BLOOD LIPID LEVELS

What about other measurements of your health status? Periodically, your family physician will check your blood lipid levels, since elevated levels are an additional risk factor for vascular problems. As demonstrated in Rita's case, blood lipid levels usually improve markedly with good diabetes management. You will probably find an annual check adequate in most instances. If your lipid levels are elevated, however, more frequent tests are required until the levels return to normal.

If, after your blood glucose levels have been normal for a while, your blood lipid levels are still elevated even though your glycosylated hemoglobin levels (hemoglobin A_{1c}) are near normal, then you may have another specific problem with blood lipids. It is not uncommon for diabetic persons to have problems with the thyroid, which may effect changes in blood lipid profiles. In any case, if your cholesterol and triglyceride levels stay high despite excellent glucose control, ask your doctor to help you find out if there is another problem leading to the elevated lipid levels. Many good drugs are now available to lower blood lipids and thereby minimize risks for heart disease in persons with diabetes.

TESTS OF KIDNEY FUNCTION

Your kidneys also reflect the state of your diabetes control. Infections should be treated immediately, and you should have your urine tested for protein. If your physician finds excess protein in your urine, this indicates that the filtering unit, the glomerulus, is not functioning properly and is "leaking" protein. You may also be given several blood tests to evaluate your kidney function, including serum creatinine and blood urea nitrogen (BUN), which measure how well your kidneys excrete waste products.

Another test that should be performed on your urine is one called a microalbuminuria test. Minor seepage of a small protein called albumin occurs early in the process of kidney damage, before the damage becomes so great as to cause a major leak of proteins from the blood into the urine. If a microalbuminuria test shows such trace amounts of albumin in the urine, it is possible to reverse or stabilize the damage before it is too late. You need to have this test if the doctor says you have "no protein" in your urine. It is possible that you have small amounts of albumin in your urine even when the protein tests show no protein. A number of drugs can help your kidneys recover and minimize the "leakiness" of proteins. The most common of these drugs are the ACE inhibitors. ACE is an abbreviation for angiotensin converting enzyme. By inhibiting this enzyme, the pressure is taken off the filtering unit, or glomerulus, of the kidney. The lower the pressure in a filter, the less likely it is to leak, and this is what happens in the kidney. Therefore, it is important to know as soon as possible if you are having problems with your kidneys since good treatments are available for the problem.

You can help prevent early problems with your kidneys by normalizing blood glucose over time. Even if problems have occurred, you can probably retard their progression with good care of your diabetes. If you are prone to recurrent kidney infections, you can test your urine with reagent strips like the ones used to test for sugar in the blood, which will tell you if you have begun another infection. This approach will enable you to start early treatment when infection does reappear. In these cases, it is often helpful to discuss with your doctor whether you should keep antibiotics on hand or even take antibiotics in a preventive fashion.

MONITORING YOUR BLOOD GLUCOSE

Your physician undoubtedly has taken intermittent blood glucose tests to monitor your diabetes control, but as both you and your doctor know, a little behavior modification on your part before the test can make the results look much better than they really might be. A more accurate indicator of your diabetes control over the last month or so would be your hemoglobin A_{1c} levels. The hemoglobin A1c test tells you and your physician whether your prescribed therapy is adequate or not since it tells what your average blood glucose has been over about the last three months.

A third area of good measure is for you to know what your blood glucose level is at a given time. Home blood glucose monitoring enables you to do this.

Before scientific advances led to home blood glucose monitoring, diabetics relied on a urine test to monitor levels. The drawback of the urine test is that the amount of glucose in the urine does not reflect the level of glucose in the blood at the moment of the test. A test may not become "positive" until glucose levels have been high for several hours.

Look at it this way. Imagine owning a car whose speedometer did not begin to register your speed until you were two or three times over the limit. You'd probably want a better speedometer—one that measured your speed accurately so that you could drive within a safe range.

A similar situation arises when you try to monitor your blood glucose with urine testing. Suppose we tell you that you will be healthy only if your blood sugar does not register outside a specific, normal range. And suppose we say you can only measure your blood glucose by urine testing. We point out that urine testing does not tell you if you're outside the normal range until you are two or three times above it. You'd probably insist on a better device to measure your blood glucose. You'd want to have the most accurate tool to verify that you are "driving" in the normal range. Home blood glucose monitoring provides you with that tool.

Blood glucose levels are measured in milligrams of sugar per deciliter of blood (mg/dl) or in millimoles (mM) in many other countries. To convert mg/dl to mM simply divide by 18. Therefore, a blood glucose level of 180 mg/dl is the same as 10 mM. Because mg/dl units are most common in the United States, we will continue to give numbers with these units. Your goal is to maintain your blood glucose before meals at between 60 mg/dl and 100 mg/dl, and not to go any higher than 150 mg/dl one hour after meals. (For simplicity, we'll drop the "mg/dl" in referring to glucose levels hereafter.)

As you know, diabetes is a condition in which the body cannot use the glucose produced by the digestion of food because it does not produce enough insulin. The level at which glucose appears in the urine—or, to be more technical, the level at which glucose spills into the urine from the kidneys—is called the renal threshold. (The word *renal* comes from the Latin *renes*, or kidneys.)

Normally the renal threshold is about 180. That's three times above the blood glucose level you need to maintain before meals. It's also much higher than the level below which you should keep after meals.

That's why you obviously can't rely on urine glucose spills to tell you that your blood sugar is low enough to ensure your well-being. Your urine will remain clear of glucose, or sugar, until your blood sugar reaches 180.

Only when you measure your blood sugar can you make appropriate judgments on your insulin and food needs. At present, this process generally requires a drop of blood. Soon "minimally invasive" approaches using smaller amounts of blood or interstitial fluid will be available. Noninvasive approaches to monitoring blood glucose are also under development in a number of laboratories.

HOW TO MONITOR YOUR BLOOD GLUCOSE AT HOME

When you monitor your blood glucose at home, you will soon become the world's expert at testing your own blood and your diabetes. At first, taking your own blood sample may sound frightening. Actually, all it involves is a tiny pinprick. Once you get a small drop of blood, you can squeeze your finger to make the drop large enough for the test.

Remember that glucose is found everywhere in the body. That's why a very tiny pinprick can be squeezed by tissue juice into a large drop of blood. The surrounding tissue juice has almost the same sugar level as the blood. The minimally invasive tests use this principle and can therefore measure the tissue juice or interstitial fluid to approximate blood sugar.

Can you use an automatic device to make sticking your finger painless? Yes—but why bother? Once you practice finger-sticking, you'll be able to do it effortlessly with minimal discomfort whatsoever.

Here's a tip that will make sticking your finger painless. Stick the side of your finger rather than the tip, where the nerves are centered. The sides of your fingers are less sensitive than the very tips. The supply of blood is also at its fullest at the sides. You can also use your insulin needle to obtain blood. These needles are smaller and thus cause less pain. Merely advance the needle until you start to feel it. It is now at a depth where there are capillaries and you can withdraw the needle and obtain a drop of blood in a relatively painless manner. Most people draw blood from the sides of the fingertips to avoid pain. The nerves, which allow pain to be felt, are more concentrated in the inner part of the finger pad (see Figure. 2.2).

Here's what you'll need for your blood glucose test:

1. A small-gauge needle, or the needle that's on your insulin syringe.
2. Test strips with a blood target on the tips.
3. A machine to read the glucose level, which may also be part of your kit.

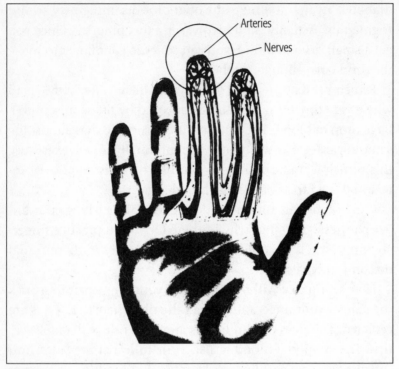

Arteries

Nerves

Figure 2.2 Arteries and Nerves of the Finger

When your glucose interacts with a substance on the glucose target portion of your test strip, the color of the pad will change or a signal will be given. Some diabetic persons just use a reagent strip and compare the changed color with a color-standard chart, which indicates the range of the glucose level.

In general, most systems still use color reagent strips. However, you may wish to consider some of the alternative methods that do not use strips. All methods still require a drop of blood, although a great deal of work is being done to find other ways of measuring blood sugar. New meter systems are available that use electrochemical ways of detecting sugar as opposed to systems that rely on enzyme-impregnated strips. In choosing which system is best for you, consider the answers to the following questions:

1. How good is the support for the system from the maker and the vendor?
2. Is there a phone number you can call if you have any problems?
3. How accurate and precise are the results? That is, can you get close to a known reference solution every time you do the test and does the value come up the same on repeated tests?
4. Is the system sufficiently portable to meet your needs?
5. If you are considering reading strips without a meter, can you tell the colors apart sufficiently to get good readings? (Many men have trouble reading the blue/green colors.)
6. Do you find the test easy to perform and does it appear foolproof?
7. Do you want a system with memory or record-keeping functions? It is often helpful to maintain a "running average" over time. This running average should agree relatively well with the results of the hemoglobin A_{1c} test.

Testing Procedure

Following are ten easy steps to follow when performing home blood glucose monitoring (Figure 2.3).

1. Position your index finger between your thumb and your middle finger.
2. Squeeze the index finger tight. You'll see the sides of

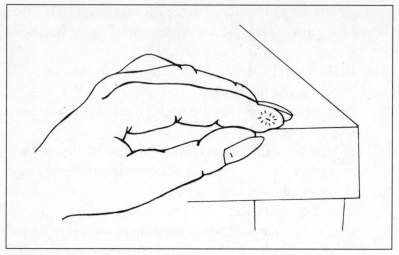

Figure 2.3 Testing Procedure

your finger "pink up," which shows you where the blood supply is best.

3. Steady your fingers against the edge of a table so you won't jolt them when you stick your finger with your other hand.

4. Poke your index finger with the needle—a teeny, tiny poke is all you need. Once you start to feel the poke, you have probably gone far enough with a small needle.

5. Release your index finger and relax.

6. Shake your hand gently and let it drop down by your side.

7. "Milk down" your index finger until you get a drop of blood.

8. Turn your finger over and allow the drop of blood to hang, and then drop it gently onto the pad of the test strip.

9. Let the machine do the rest or read the directions on your reagent strip bottle to see how long you should leave the blood on the strip.

10. Always be sure you are accurate by comparing your results with a standardized method referenced to a laboratory method when you are first beginning to test as well as periodically thereafter.

Testing Without a Meter

In addition to measuring your blood glucose with a glucose meter, you may want to try doing the test with another system that does not require a meter. This type of system is based on test strips that you can read yourself. Before you switch to this system, you have to test your ability to use it accurately. Compare your reading of the visually readable test pad with your meter's reading of a test strip. Do this over and over again until you're sure you can accurately read a test strip that does not involve a meter. Then you will be free to test your blood glucose levels without the meter.

The best part of self-monitoring your blood glucose with visually readable test strips is that you can do the test more easily anywhere—at home or in public, for example, at a restaurant. And after you obtain a drop of blood, you can have your test result in one or two minutes—and with it that feeling of security that comes from knowing you're right on target. If you're not, the test will let you know whether you have to take a bit more insulin, delay your meal for a while, or eat right away.

With careful monitoring, you can have near normal blood sugar, known as euglycemia. Keeping blood sugar normal is like walking a tightrope—but it gets easier the more you practice.

Choosing a System

We have found that most of the available systems perform well and are becoming more reasonably priced. Companies are now trying to make meters which will be even more suitable for patients. You should make certain before purchasing any instrument that supplies and service are readily available. Discuss your needs in detail with a diabetes professional, pharmacist, or company representative, and ask for a demonstration of the instrument before purchasing. In most cases, purchase of the instrument and supplies is a reimbursable expense under a medical insurance policy. Reagent strips that can be read visually with satisfactory accuracy are also available. If you read the strips visually, you must be careful to train your eye with a standard reference. If you have problems in color perception, stay with the meter system.

It is extremely important that you feel comfortable with the system before you use its results to adjust your insulin dosage. Comprehensive instructions are provided by the centers that sell the glucose meters and you can usually master the operation within a day.

Nervousness about taking your blood sample may make it hard to get your blood to flow smoothly, but this will come with practice. If you have any problems or questions with the system, ask a health care professional, pharmacist, or company representative to help you. It is important that you use the instrument accurately because the measurements you obtain will determine what you do in terms of medication, food, and exercise and provide the key to your success in maintaining good control.

Whenever a medical laboratory test is performed, two issues must be addressed: accuracy and precision. These two concepts are also very important for the person performing home glucose monitoring. Therefore an explanation is in order.

Let's use archery as an example. If you are accurate in shooting your arrows, you will hit the bull's-eye every time. The arrows may not all hit exactly at the same point, but they will be within the bull's-eye. Likewise, accuracy in a laboratory test means hitting the true mark or goal every time. The way to make sure that your values are accurate is to have a reference or standard where you know the true value and make sure you get that value. Therefore, most companies provide a standard or calibration solution so that the accuracy of a given blood glucose self-monitoring procedure can be tested.

To continue the archery analogy, let's say that you do not always hit the center of the target every time but you always place your arrows in the same spot. That is precision, hitting the same place with every try. Precision is also extremely important in blood glucose monitoring. If you know your equipment gives you the same reading every time, then you can rely on those numbers to make judgments. If you cannot get the same number, then your blood glucose monitoring system has problems.

What is a reasonable precision range? Generally, the systems can be made to perform within 10 percent. That is, if a sample is run over and over again, the values should fall within 10 percent of each other. Values with a precision of 20 percent can be tolerated, but greater deviations should definitely be corrected.

Therefore, when performing home blood glucose monitoring you will want to reference your machine to another system such as the one in a laboratory, physician's office, or pharmacy to make sure the values are accurate. You will also want to make sure that your machine is precise by running a given solution or sample over and over again to check whether the readings are consistent. Each blood glucose monitoring system should have a way of determining accuracy and precision. Ask your representative for the best way to check your system.

HOW DOES HOME MONITORING HELP YOU?

After a week of monitoring your blood glucose levels, and with the results of the HbA$_{1c}$ test your physician has given you, you can begin to get an idea of how well your diabetes is being controlled. For best results, you should time your blood glucose measurements around your meals. Take one blood glucose measurement before each meal and a second one about an hour after you have started eating. This will approximate your highest and lowest measurements of the day. If you test yourself before and after all three meals during the day, the sum of the measurements should add up to about 600 for an average blood glucose of 100 mg/dl. This sum has been found to correlate well with both hemoglobin A$_{1c}$, when it is maintained over time, and a twenty-four-hour assessment of blood glucose values.

It is also often helpful to measure blood glucose at around 3:00 in the morning, when you are most vulnerable to low blood glucose. This way you can prevent yourself from going too low. If for some reason your blood glucose is high at this time, you can also learn to "touch up" with regular insulin so you can "fix" your fasting blood glucose and start the next day right.

Another time to test is when you feel "funny." The body only has a certain number of ways to respond to internal and external stress—rapid heart rate, sweat, sick feeling in the stomach, headache, etc. Therefore it is often difficult to know whether you have a high or low sugar problem, are getting the flu, have worked out to hard, or are falling in love. When in doubt, check your blood sugar!

Here's where the fun begins. You can measure what a given food portion or insulin dosage does for you. You can also evaluate the results of a particular activity or stress situation. You can find out whether your present regimen is adequate to maintain control or requires some adjusting. You will see what happens when you get excited or depressed. In essence, you become more in touch with your feelings and how they affect your blood glucose levels. *You* control the situation and can plan accordingly.

You should settle for no less than the near-normal blood glucose range of 50–150 mg/dl. There may be times, however, when you are out of this range. You now have the ability to measure where you are and will learn to respond appropriately. You need no longer fear the unknown. You should measure your blood glucose when you feel "funny," because this may indicate a high or low blood glucose level. You may be surprised to find that many times you are actually hypoglycemic when you feel "hyper" and vice versa. As times goes on, you will be able to identify more closely what feelings accurately coincide with a given blood glucose level. Knowing your blood glucose level, then, is the first step in ridding yourself of the fear of diabetes itself. Another thing you will notice as good control is achieved is that you are better able to sense when you are low because you have trained yourself for "hypoglycemic awareness" and the consequences of low glucose are less severe. Persons who keep their glucose in the normal range usually first sense hypoglycemia with a tingling or "funny" sensation in and around the mouth, whereas persons who are out of control don't realize they are low until they perspire, get ravenously hungry, or have other symptoms described later.

Keeping Records

Another aid to good medical care is to keep good records. You should keep a daily diary to enter how you feel, what you eat, your blood glucose and urine ketone measurements when you are sick, exercise, activities, and any other comments you may have. You should note what you do and the time you do it so

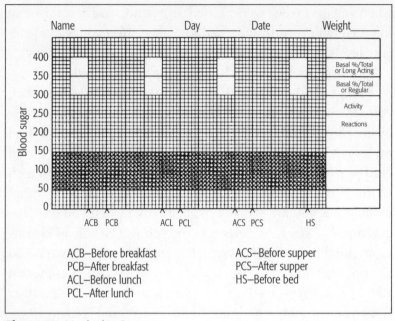

Figure 2.4 Monitoring System

that you can start to learn how your diabetes affects you and what you can do about it.

You'll find that your diary becomes an invaluable record. You can learn at what blood glucose level you begin to spill glucose into your urine. You can find out how much a given amount of insulin lowered your blood glucose and what certain foods did to your blood glucose. Having this record allows you to go back and discuss the problems that bothered you during the week with your physician, other health care professionals, family, or friends. Having a team work on problems usually leads to solutions more quickly, so build your own team as soon as possible and keep it going. As you learn more about yourself and your diabetes, you will find that many things that had no explanation at first become more easily understood in retrospect. By measuring what you are doing and keeping good records, you will soon become the master of your diabetes.

Figure 2.4 is a form that we often use to initiate diabetic persons into home blood glucose monitoring. The goal is to get all blood glucose levels into the "normal" range (shaded area). When you use a chart such as this, you can accurately record exercise, meal times, meal carbohydrate content, medication, insulin type, insulin shot time, and hypoglycemic reactions. With the information recorded, you'll be able to see changes in patterns. And when you see changes, you can make the necessary adjustments to get your patterns back to "normal."

3

Diabetes Medications

There are two means of drug delivery whereby the high blood glucose level of a diabetic person can be improved. The first is with oral hypoglycemic agents, also called antidiabetic drugs, and the second is with the use of insulin by injection. These two means of drug delivery will be discussed separately.

ORAL HYPOGLYCEMIC MEDICATIONS

Only those diabetic persons with some functioning pancreas can get along with the oral medications. Remember, the definition of type 1 diabetes is complete loss of pancreatic function. Thus, the oral agents are not appropriate for the type 1 patient. These patients require insulin. It is unfortunate that insulin is not available in pill form, but gastric (stomach) juices are so acidic that insulin taken orally is quickly digested and thus does not get into the bloodstream. That is why insulin needs to be injected or delivered by implanted or genetically manipulated cells that secrete insulin.

Type 2 patients, who have some pancreas function but who do not use their own insulin efficiently, can benefit from oral agents. The oral agents not only coax the person's pancreas to try harder to secrete more insulin, but also make the available insulin more effective in burning sugar in the bloodstream and in stimulating cells to take up glucose. Another way oral agents can help is by preventing the breakdown of sugars in the gut so that they are not absorbed or are at least absorbed more slowly.

One available class of oral agents in the United States is called *sulfonylurea*. When these drugs were used as "sulfa antibiotics" during World War II, it was noticed that some patients became hypoglycemic (had low blood sugar levels). The drugs have been improved over the last forty-five years. Now we have second-generation sulfonylurea agents that are able to lower blood sugar as well as the first-generation agents, and these newer pills have only about one-hundredth the possibility of causing dangerous side effects.

Table 3.1 lists the oral agents available in the United States, along with the doses usually prescribed and how long they last.

If you are taking an oral agent, you should determine what effect these drugs have on your blood glucose. Measure your blood glucose before breakfast and one hour after each meal. The before-breakfast blood test will tell you whether the pill you took the night before is strong enough to last until morning. Usually glyburide is effective at keeping the wake-up morning blood sugar in check. Sometimes a sulfonylurea drug will work better if taken twice a day even if once a day dosing is stated as sufficient. Each person handles food and drugs a little differently and the key is to find the best dose and frequency for us.

The after-meal checks not only tell you whether you have been on the mark for your meal plan, but also whether your dose of medication is strong enough. Short acting drugs are better to take before each meal as they are generally designed to keep the

Table 3.1 Oral Hypoglycemia Agents Available in the United States

Name of Drug	Highest Dose (mg)	Duration of Action (hrs)
First Generation of Sulfonylurea Drugs		
Tolbutamide	2,000	6
Chlorpropamide	500	24
Tolazamide	1,000	12
Second Generation of Sulfonylurea Drugs		
Glyburide		
Long and short acting	15	16
Glipzide		
Long and short acting	40	12
Glimepiride	8	24
Other Insulin Secretion Enhancers		
Repaglinide*	?	?
Insulin Sensitizing Agents		
Metformin	2,500	24
Troglitazone	600	24
Starch Blocking Agents		
Acarbose	100 (before meals)	4
Migilitol*	?	4

*Not yet available

after-meal blood glucose in check.

As Table 3.1 shows, several types of oral agents are available. Each has certain advantages and disadvantages. Because each type of oral hypoglycemic drug works in a different way, they may often be used in combination(s) to increasingly improve glucose levels. In general, it is wise to start each drug separately and determine its effect. If you tolerate the first drug well and get some benefit, then consider your next step. If the glucose levels achieved are not what you would like, consider adding the second drug. Remember, for each drug you add you not only increase the chance of a drug reaction but also increase the chances of a drug interaction—a side effect from the combination of drugs that would not occur with either one alone.

Sulfonylurea Drugs

The sulfonylurea drugs have been in use for the longest period of time and therefore are "tried and true." They work, in general, by increasing insulin output from the beta cells of the pancreas. They also have other effects. Nevertheless, if there is no insulin available in your pancreas (as in type 1 diabetes), these pills will not be useful for you and you will need insulin. Likewise, if your pancreas is becoming exhausted and unable to secrete much more insulin, these drugs will no longer be able to help you. This failure of sulfonylurea drugs often occurs in people who have taken them for a long period of time. Often after a "vacation" from the drug, the pancreas will be rested during intensive insulin treatment and the oral agents can be used again.

The sulfonylurea drugs are grouped into first and second generation. The first generation drugs have been around the longest. They tend to require higher doses and bind more avidly to carrier proteins. For this reason, they are more apt to interfere with other drugs you might be taking (a drug-drug interaction as discussed above). Therefore, most physicians favor the second generation agents. These agents appear fairly comparable and come in short and long acting formulations. If your primary problem is that your morning glucose is high, you would probably want a longer acting drug so that its effect will last over night. If your primary problem is a high after-meal glucose, you might want to start with a shorter acting preparation. All the sulfonylurea drugs stimulate insulin to be secreted and therefore the main side effect is the potential for hypoglycemia. The potential for low blood sugars can be worsened after a few drinks of alcohol. One of the most vulnerable times for low blood sugar is in the middle of the night when the hormones that protect the body from low blood sugars are at their lowest. When in doubt, check your blood sugar at 3:00 A.M. when starting these new agents or after exposure to alcohol. Initial reports suggest that glimepiride may be less likely to cause hypoglycemia but the experience with this drug is still limited. Sulfonylurea compounds bind to a receptor on the beta-cell and glimepiride binds to a different protein or binding area than the others. Whether a different binding site has advantages or whether it can be used in combination with other sulfonylurea agents remains in doubt.

The sulfonylurea drugs have become accepted as being quite safe and effective, but their use in patients with heart disease is controversial. While the drugs act by inhibiting potassium channels that induce the release of insulin in the pancreas, they also inhibit similar ATP (energy compound) sensitive potassium channels in the heart. These channels can help protect the heart from injury due to lack of oxygen during a heart attack. Therefore, the use of these types of drugs in persons at high risk for a heart attack is being questioned.

Insulin Secretion Enhancers

Other drugs that are not sulfonylurea compounds also enhance insulin secretion. Repaglinide is the first of these compounds to be marketed in Europe and will soon be available in the United States as well. It binds to the same site as the sulfonylurea drugs as well as others that also appear to result in an increase in insulin secretion. It seems to work more quickly and may be more potent than sulfonylurea-type drugs. A number of similar drugs will also be coming on the market. Again, whether these types of drugs (the meglitinides) have advantages or can be used in combination with other drugs remains to be determined.

Insulin Sensitizing Drugs

In addition to drugs that push extra insulin out of the pancreas, drugs are also available to make tissues more sensitive to insulin. The two primary sites for the action of these types of insulin sensitizing agents are the liver and the muscles. The liver is in charge of storing glucose and releasing it into the bloodstream. The muscle is a major site for taking up glucose so that it can be available for energy during exercise.

Metformin is a drug that has been used in Europe for more than thirty years and was introduced to the United States more recently. It is useful because it not only improves glucose levels but also has an effect on appetite. Persons taking metformin tend to lose weight whereas other glucose lowering agents and insulin are often associated with weight gain. While the duration of action of metformin in lowering glucose is fairly long, the drug effect on appetite is most apparent if it is taken before meals.

The drug may have some side effects on intestinal function, such as nausea and diarrhea. For this reason, it is helpful to begin with a low dose and slowly build up to the best dose over time. If the starting dose leads to side effects, the dose can be lowered until you become accustomed to the drug. With the right dose, most persons can get used to the drug in a way that allows the benefits to become apparent without the side effects. Another side effect of metformin is lactic acidosis. This kind of acid can build up in the bloodstream if a person has ongoing liver or kidney disease or if a person is in heart failure. Lactic acid can also build up in the blood after alcohol use. Therefore, when starting the drug, liver and kidney function tests should be performed and followed. In addition, the drug should be stopped if you need to be hospitalized since tests or procedures are often performed that may adversely affect kidney and liver function, or the person may be admitted to the hospital with heart problems. For safety reasons, it is best to stop metformin and avoid any potential problems by replacing it with insulin. Nevertheless, when given properly, metformin is an extremely useful and safe drug. It is also of great use in combination with other drugs or insulin.

Troglitazone is a newer insulin sensitizing drug. The primary site of action appears to be on muscle where the drug stimulates uptake of glucose. It also has some effect on the liver, which is the primary site of toxicity for the drug. Liver function tests are monitored at least annually for persons taking troglitazone. If the liver function tests go up, the drug is stopped. Troglitazone and metformin appear to have similar strength in lowering glucose. They also appear to be additive in their effects. Troglitazone is also used frequently with insulin if it is not effective enough by itself. Like metformin, it may take one to two months before the best effect of troglitazone on blood glucose levels is realized. Troglitazone is generally administered with a meal but it does not have the appetite suppressant properties of metformin. Other drugs in the same family as troglitazone (the thiazolidinediones) are currently being developed and may be less toxic to the liver. Nausea, vomiting, abdominal pain, loss of appetite, dark urine, jaundice, and fatigue can all be signs of liver disease.

Starch Blocking Agents

Starch blockers are also useful glucose lowering agents, especially for persons who have trouble with high blood glucose after meals. They block and delay the absorption of sugars from starch. Because they are not absorbed themselves, they are relatively safe although persons may initially complain of gas or intestinal disturbances. Again, persistence pays off and with careful adjustments of the dose or by taking simethacone to absorb the gas, most people can use these agents effectively. These types of drugs are seldom of use by themselves but are often useful along with other drugs in maintaining better glucose levels after meals.

Managing Type 2 Diabetes

The first line of approach to type 2 diabetes is often diet and exercise. Next, choose an appropriate first line drug. If you have high insulin and/or C-peptide levels, that means your pancreas is working hard but you are resistant to the insulin you are making. In this case, it might be worth starting with an insulin sensitizing agent. By checking your sugars before and after you eat, you will know if you are winning with your approach. If your sugars are still not fixed, then you may want to add another drug to help your pancreas make more insulin (a sulfonylurea), another insulin sensitizing drug (for example, add troglitazone to metformin), a drug to lower after meal sugars (a starch blocker), or take a little insulin to help out the other medications. At each step of the way, work with your doctor and health care team to define what you want a drug to accomplish, what side effects or drug interactions might occur, how much time you are going to wait for the effect, and what you will do next.

Do not ignore insulin. It is still the best drug for lowering blood glucose and is amazingly safe if used correctly. If your blood glucose levels are not improved by oral agents, the next step is to add insulin. A bedtime dose of NPH or intermediate acting insulin (see below) is a helpful addition. If a person wakes up with high blood glucose, then even if the level does not go much higher with meals, the diabetes is still "out of control" (see Figure 3.1). Having a high morning blood glucose in and of itself can make you resistant to insulin. If the blood glucose is normal at the waking hour, then oral medications have a chance to keep the blood sugar normal (see Figure 3.1). This is why "fixing the fasting" or wake-up sugar is generally the first step in diabetes management.

During illness or other times of stress, it will help to know your blood glucose levels even if you are taking oral agents. At these times you may "break through" oral medication and then require insulin therapy. You may also want to know your urine ketone levels to make sure acid is not building up during these times of extra stress. But no matter what kind of diabetes you have or what steps you use to control it, it is always important to measure what you are doing.

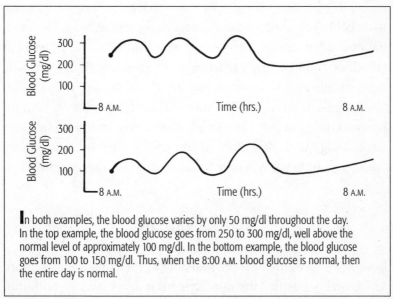

In both examples, the blood glucose varies by only 50 mg/dl throughout the day. In the top example, the blood glucose goes from 250 to 300 mg/dl, well above the normal level of approximately 100 mg/dl. In the bottom example, the blood glucose goes from 100 to 150 mg/dl. Thus, when the 8:00 A.M. blood glucose is normal, then the entire day is normal.

Figure 3.1 The Effect of Oral Medications on Blood Glucose Levels

How often should you measure your blood glucose if you have type 2 diabetes, and how can you find out if your medications are working? Average blood glucose in a person with type 2 diabetes tends to correlate well with the fasting or early-morning blood glucose level. In general, this value should be around 100. Therefore, the fasting level should be measured daily to make sure you are not "sneaking out of control." The major problem in type 2 diabetes tends to be with food. Your major task will be to identify which foods affect your blood sugar adversely and then to avoid or cut back on these foods. The peak blood glucose occurs forty-five to ninety minutes after you begin your meal. Therefore, to check the effect of food on blood sugar, you should check one hour after you begin the meal. This will keep you honest in terms of the kinds of meals you are eating. Most people have problems with too much carbohydrate for breakfast and too much food for dinner. Thus you may want to monitor these meals fairly often. Restaurant foods often have hidden carbohydrates that are not apparent from looking at your plate so check after trying new menus to be better prepared the next time. Finally, you will want to check your blood glucose whenever you feel "funny" or ill. Illness can raise blood glucose even when you have not eaten, and you may need insulin to tide you through an illness despite the fact that you have been doing well on your oral medication or on your fitness and diet plan (see Chapter 10). Conversely, you may find yourself drifting low during illness without realizing it because you are "sick." In summary, when in doubt, check out your glucose level.

YOUR INSULIN

Several kinds of insulins are available in the United States. Since 1975, highly purified insulins have been developed. In addition, thanks to new technology, human insulin is now available. Most recently, "designer insulins" are being developed and have reached the marketplace. When insulin first became commercially available in 1922, it was obtained mostly from animals, mainly pigs and cows. Animal insulins have a slightly different chemical structure than does human insulin. Although animal insulins do lower the blood sugar in a human being, they can cause some adverse reactions. These reactions range from mild skin problems with redness and swelling at the injection site, to the formation of antibodies that weaken the potency of the insulin, to major allergic reactions that can even be fatal. Human insulin is now commercially available, and it is recommended for children, pregnant women, and patients with manifestations of animal insulin allergy. The designer insulins use human insulin as the starting point, and then through genetic engineering, change one or more of the building blocks so that the insulin functions in a more desirable way. For example, lispro insulin absorbs much faster from the injection site than even regular insulin. *Lis* and *pro* stand for the building blocks that have been rearranged in the human insulin molecule to make it absorb much more quickly. Lispro is used right before meals. It is so rapid in its action that it is still effective even if injected after the meal. For this reason, it is especially useful if you are not sure what you might eat or if your child is a finicky or unpredictable eater. Just wait and see what is eaten, and then you can decide how much lispro you need to cover the food consumed.

Two popular families of insulins are the NPH family and the Lente family (see Table 3.2), both of which can be made from animal sources or as human insulin.

The NPH Family

The NPH family consists of three insulins: Regular, NPH, and PZI. Regular is a short-acting insulin. It starts to act at 1 to 2 hours, is strongest at 3 to 4 hours, and is gone at 6 hours (see Figure 3.2.)

Table 3.2 Action of Available Insulins

Family	Type	Onset (hrs)	Peak (hrs)	Duration (hrs)
NPH	Regular	1½–2	3–4	6
	NPH	4	8–12	18
	PZI	4	18–24	36
Lente	Semilente	1½–2	3–4	6
	Lente	4	8–12	18–24
	Ultralente	4	(no peak if given properly—lasts 18 hours)	
Designer insulins	Lispro	¼	1–2	3

NPH is an intermediate-acting insulin. NPH stands for Neutral Protamine Hagedorn. It is named after H.C. Hagedorn, a Danish physician who, in the 1930s, prolonged the action of the quick insulins by adding neutral protamine. The result is an insulin that starts to act at 4 hours, is strongest at 8 to 12 hours, and is essentially gone by 18 hours.

PZI is the longest-acting insulin in the NPH family. The letters stand for Protamine Zinc Insulin. PZI starts to work at 4 hours, peaks from 18 to 24 hours, and lasts 36 hours. I prefer the NPH family of insulin because in each person the onset, peak, and duration of the insulin tends to be more predictable and consistent in most people. Lispro insulin is also very reliable and useful for fixing the after meal sugars. It can be calculated just like regular insulin but needs to be given without a "lag time." It is also quickly utilized so there is no need for a snack after its use to match with leftover insulin after the mealtime carbohydrates were covered. It is possible to mix and match insulin families. For the purposes of discussion, we will keep the families together.

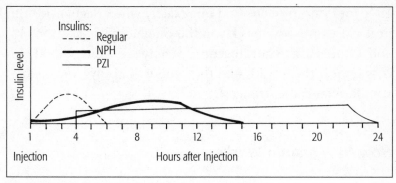

Figure 3.2 The NPH Family of Insulins: Onset, Peak, Duration

How Regular Insulin Works

Let's start with the short-acting insulin, the Regular. The best use of Regular insulin is before a meal, to "touch up" at 3:00 to 4:00 A.M., or in an insulin pump. Because of its peak in about three hours, it helps you to utilize food (convert it to energy). It also prevents blood glucose from going too high after a meal. For example, if you plan to inject Regular insulin before breakfast, check your blood glucose before the injection and then every fifteen minutes afterward. As soon as your blood glucose falls fifteen points, eat breakfast. You now know your personal "lag time" for Regular. This lag time is generally one-half to one hour for Regular.

The lag time between the injection of Regular insulin and the falling glucose level is the time it takes for the insulin to get into your bloodstream. This lag time is referred to as the *onset* of your insulin. Once you have determined your personal lag time, you will know exactly how long to wait after an injection of Regular before you can eat your meal.

The *peak* of your Regular insulin occurs three to four hours after your injection. To find our exactly when Regular insulin peaks in your body, check your blood glucose at 2, 2½, 3, 3½, and 4 hours after your injection. Merely see which blood glucose level is the lowest, and then you will always know when your Regular is the strongest.

How NPH Insulin Works

You are probably taking NPH insulin with your Regular, and therefore you must learn when NPH is strongest in your body. To find out, try this experiment. Measure your blood glucose 4, 5, 6, 7, 8, 9, and 10 hours after your injection. If you faithfully do all of these blood glucose checks, you should be able to chart your NPH insulin strength so that it's similar to the heavy line (NPH) in Figure 3.2. You'll also find out that NPH works in you pretty predictably.

Mimicking Normal Pancreatic Secretions of Insulin

The best way to use this NPH family of insulin is to mix and match the NPH and Regular to mimic normal pancreatic secretions of insulin.

What's normal? The normal pancreas puts out a little insulin all the time—even when you are not eating (see Figure 3.3). This low-dose insulin secretion prevents the glucose stored in the liver from being released into the bloodstream. If you do not maintain a low level of insulin in your bloodstream all the time, sugar stores are unleashed and blood glucose levels rise. The levels may actually go higher than you could achieve if you ate pure table sugar. This is why sugars may rise overnight even if you have not eaten anything before bed or during the night. Thus the normal pancreas secretes "basal insulin" levels and "bolus" or food associated insulin.

In addition to putting out a little insulin all the time, the normal pancreas puts out more insulin before each meal or snack, the bolus. As a person gets hungry and prepares to eat, the pancreas starts to put out the additional insulin even before the first morsel is taken. This premeal secretion of insulin is called the cephalic phase. The word *cephalic* means "pertaining to the head," and the term suggests that just thinking about food causes the pancreas to prepare for doing its part in the digestive process.

In general, the normal pattern of insulin secretion varies according to the size of the meal or whether a meal is in fact eaten or skipped.

Attaining Round-the-Clock Insulin Coverage with NPH and Regular Insulin

To mimic the pattern of normal pancreatic secretions as shown in Figure 3.3, a long-acting insulin must be injected. PZI could be used, but recently PZI has not been favored, partly because it seems to stimulate the body's immune system. Instead, two injections of NPH are used to supply the basal insulin and keep the blood glucose level normal between meals. Standard usage includes one injection in the morning and one before bed. If your NPH insulin peaks in eight to nine hours and becomes weak after that, an injection at 8:00 A.M. will work until 4:00 or 5:00 P.M. From 4:00 P.M. to bedtime, however, you will not have enough insulin to keep the liver from releasing glucose. As shown in Figure 3.4, a gap in insulin levels develops between 4:00 and 5:00 P.M. and at 11:00 P.M.

What do you do to cover this gap? An injection of Regular

insulin before dinner will cover dinner and fill the gap with enough insulin to hold you until bedtime, when you will take an injection of NPH (see Figure 3.5). Thus, you would have around the clock coverage with insulin.

Of course, you probably also want to eat breakfast and lunch. To cover a breakfast meal, you would take Regular with your NPH before breakfast, as shown in Figure 3.6.

What about lunch? You have two choices here. You could add a lunchtime injection of Regular, or you could increase the NPH at breakfast to be strong enough to cover the midday meal.

The advantages of making the NPH strong enough to cover the midday meal is that you are keeping your daily injections to three, as follows:

1. NPH and Regular mixed together before breakfast
2. Regular before dinner
3. NPH before bed

The disadvantage of this system is that if you do not eat lunch on time or if you do not eat enough lunch, you are at the mercy of your already injected NPH; therefore, you have no choice but to eat and to eat on time.

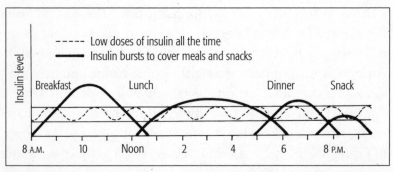

Figure 3.3 Pattern of Normal Pancreatic Secretion of Insulin in a Basal or Resting State and Around Meals

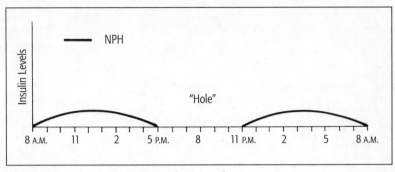

Figure 3.4 Using Two Injections of NPH Daily

If you want to skip lunch, keep your NPH dose before breakfast just at the right level to keep your blood sugar normal when you are not eating. Then if you skip lunch you can stay normal until dinner, or you can have the freedom to delay lunch. If you do delay lunch, you must add a fourth injection of Regular to cover the lunch meal.

Figure 3.7 shows how coverage is attained using three injections of insulin a day. Figure 3.8 shows coverage using four injections a day. Notice how the insulin patterns in Figures 3.7 and 3.8 match the pattern of normal pancreatic secretions of insulin as shown in Figure 3.3 on page 54.

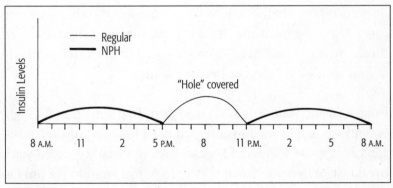

Figure 3.5 Using Regular to Fill 5:00 P.M. to 11:00 P.M. Gap

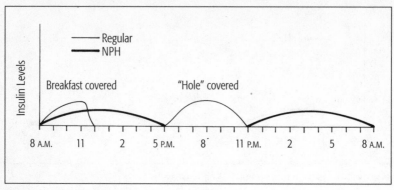

Figure 3.6 Using Regular to Cover Breakfast

Determining Your Doses

In order to find out how much insulin you need for your between-meal doses of NPH and your mealtime doses of Regular, you must check your blood glucose levels at least seven times a day.

Your check just before breakfast gives you two pieces of information. First, it tells you whether your bedtime injection of NPH is just right to keep you normal overnight. In addition, the before-breakfast check tells you how much Regular insulin to take for breakfast. To appropriately mimic the normal pancreas, this prebreakfast Regular insulin must be increased or decreased depending on whether you wake up too low, too high, or just right. Not only must the Regular insulin be just right to cover breakfast, but it may need to be increased or decreased depending on your blood glucose before the meal.

Using a Sliding Scale. You can create a sliding scale that will tell you how much Regular insulin you need for your meals. For instance, suppose 6 units of Regular insulin usually covered your breakfast. When you woke up too low, you would take only 4

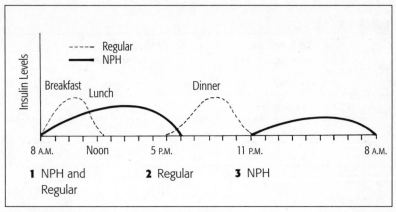

Figure 3.7 Using Three Injections of Insulin Daily

units; when you woke up slightly high, you'd take 8 units; and if you woke up higher, you'd take 10 units (see Table 3.3).

Now, how is your individual dosage determined? Your ideal dose of Regular for each meal depends on two variables: your body weight and the carbohydrates of the meal you are about to eat.

If you are not insulin "resistant" or "sensitive" and need total insulin replacement, your doctor will write down an insulin

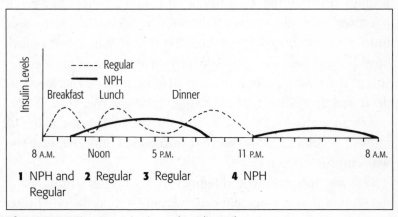

Figure 3.8 Using Four Injections of Insulin Daily

TABLE 3.3 Sliding Scale for Insulin

Prebreakfast Blood Sugar Level	Amount of Regular Insulin to Take
Under 70	4 units
70–100	6
100–140	8
Over 140	10

dose based on your body weight at about 0.6 units per kilogram. For example, suppose a patient named Ann weighs 132 pounds, or 60 kilograms in the metric system. She'll probably be taking 36 units of insulin daily ($60 \times 0.6 = 36$).

The dose is divided into three injections a day, with two-thirds of the total taken in the morning. Thus, Ann's morning injection totals 24 units. That's two-thirds of the 36 units she requires. The total morning dose (24 units in Ann's case) is divided into two parts NPH to one part Regular. Thus, Ann's 24 units are roughly divided into 16 units of NPH and 8 units of Regular. (In cases where the numbers do not divide evenly, fractions of units are not counted.) Ann takes her morning injection before breakfast, but after she has taken a blood glucose reading. As a result of the reading, her 8 units of Regular may be increased or decreased depending on her waking blood glucose. Thus, if Ann wakes up with an 8:00 A.M. blood glucose of 110, she takes 10 units of Regular (2 more than her calculated 8 units because she woke up slightly high).

Let's see how Ann would figure this out on her sliding scale. Remember that her normal dose would be 16 units NPH plus 8 Regular for a total of 24. Thus her sliding scale would look like Table 3.4.

TABLE 3.4 Sample Morning Sliding Scale

Prebreakfast Blood Sugar Level	Amount of Regular Insulin to Take
Under 70	6 units
70–100	8
100–140	10
Over 140	12

On the morning Ann wakes up with an 8:00 A.M. blood glucose of 110, she looks at the insulin amount corresponding to a blood sugar range of 100–140. The amount is 10 units of Regular, to which is added 16 units of NPH to make a new total of 26. The glucose targets of a sliding scale may vary depending on your optimum glucose levels, which are decided upon by you and your health care team.

Ann is generally allowed to take no more than 4 extra units of Regular (in her case, no more than 12 units total) even if she wakes up extremely high. Instead, she is told to wait to eat until her blood glucose falls below 120. This could mean that she will need to skip a meal, but that's better than having her take too much of Regular, which may open up the risk of a severe insulin reaction. In addition, eating on top of a high blood glucose level only makes the sugar go higher. Since Ann's goal is normal blood glucose, it is more important for her to conquer her high sugar than to eat. Indeed, eating when the blood sugar is high only wastes the food since excess sugar will "spill" into the urine anyway.

To ensure that the insulin you take to cover breakfast is strong enough to get you through the meal, you must take a blood sugar reading one hour after the meal. People absorb food at different rates, but for each person the absorption pattern is relatively consistent. A mixed meal (one with carbohydrate, protein, and fat) causes your blood glucose to be at its highest about one hour after beginning the meal.

Now you understand why the best times to measure your blood glucose level is before a meal (to know how your basal dose is doing and how much Regular to take for the meal) and one hour after a meal (to ensure the Regular was strong enough for the meal).

Now back to our patient. Ann has chosen the three-injection-a-day plan. This means she checks her blood glucose level one hour after lunch to see if her morning NPH was strong enough.

Ann also checks her blood sugar before dinner. This check serves as a double-check on the morning NPH dose, and it allows for the dinner Regular to be adjusted. In Ann's case, her dinner Regular is one-sixth of her total daily insulin requirement, or 6 units (36 ÷ 6 = 6). Ann's sliding scale at dinner would look like Table 3.5. Ann's NPH dose before bed is also one-sixth of her total insulin requirement, or 6 units of NPH.

Checking Blood Glucose Seven Times a Day Let's take a look at the record that Ann keeps of her insulin checks. It shows when and why she takes a reading. Her check always corresponds to a food peak or an insulin peak. Her check may tell Ann whether her food and insulin match or whether she should take more of her Regular or NPH. She makes seven checks a day, as in Table 3.6

There you have it. Ann takes three injections a day (NPH and Regular at 8:00 A.M.; Regular at 5:00 P.M.; and NPH at 11:00 P.M.). She's taking a total of four insulins daily (two NPH and two Regular) and eating three meals. That means she needs seven blood glucose readings: four to check the peaks of insulin and three to check the peaks of food.

TABLE 3.5 Sample Dinner Sliding Scale

Prebreakfast Blood Sugar Level	Amount of Regular Insulin to Take
Under 70	6 (2 less than calculated)
70–100	6
100–140	8 (2 more than calculated)
Over 140	10 (4 more than calculated)

The Lente Family

The second family of insulins that are widely used in the United States is the Lente family (see Table 3.1 for summary). Here the insulin action is regulated by crystal size. Smaller crystals get into the bloodstream faster; larger crystals get in slower. The family consists of *Semilente* (small crystals) similar in action to Regular; and *Ultralente,* larger crystals that confer an action similar to PZI.

Lente is a combination of small crystals (Semilente) and huge crystals (Ultralente). Lente is not an intermediate-size crystal, so its action profile is not quite similar to that of NPH. Lente has a glucose lowering peak or "punch" from the Semilente component and a punch from the Ultralente component. In addition, the two combine into a third punch in eight to twelve hours. These punches are not always predictable and depend upon crystal breakdown time. Thus it is sometimes difficult to fine-tune control with Lente insulin.

A Marriage of Two Insulin Families

A very good cross-match of families occurs, however, from the marriage of the Ultralente insulin from the Lente family with

TABLE 3.6 A Patient's Seven Daily Checks

Time	Blood Sugar	Insulin or Food	Comment
8:00 A.M.	110	16 units NPH 10 units Regular	I need 2 more units of Regular because of my high blood sugar. To fix my fasting level, I will increase my NPH before bed by 2 units.
10:00 A.M. (1 hour after breakfast)	135	20 grams of carbohydrate in breakfast	Breakfast and insulin matched.
11:30 A.M.	68	Peak of Regular from breakfast	I need milk to take the edge off my Regular "punch."
1:30 P.M.	140	50 grams of carbohydrate in lunch	Perfectly matched.
5:00 P.M.	60	5 units Regular	I am low, so I need 2 units less NPH before breakfast than calculated. I will add an afternoon snack to prevent this low tomorrow.
7:00 P.M. (1 hour after dinner)	160	60 grams of carbohydrate in dinner	I like dinner, so rather than cutting down on carbohydrates for dinner, I shall increase my insulin for tomorrow's dinner by 2 units.My scale will then be:
			Predinner Blood Sugar — *Insulin* Under 70 — 6 70–100 — 8 100–140 — 10 Over 140 — 12
8:30 P.M.	90	Peak of Regular from dinner	I need more carbohydrate at dinner so that I do not go too low here, so I have room for more Regular to cover dinner tomorrow.

the Regular insulin from the NPH family. This combination of insulins most nearly mimics normal pancreatic secretions of insulin. The between-meal glucose levels are kept normal with the Ultralente, and the meals are covered by Regular. This system requires three injections a day but actually gives the freedom of the four-injection plan described previously (see Figure 3.8 on page 57). A mixture of Ultralente and Regular is taken before breakfast. Lunch is covered by Regular insulin. The long-acting Ultralente is given with the dinner Regular and lasts until the next morning's breakfast injection. No injection is needed at bedtime. Ultralente has an onset of action four hours after the injection and has a sustained slow action of eighteen hours. This "square wave" is seen only when the Ultralente is perfectly calculated to deliver just enough insulin to maintain normal blood glucose when a person does not eat (see Figure 3.9). If too much Ultralente is injected, then Ultralente, too, delivers a punch and the duration of action is prolonged up to thirty-six hours, depending on the size of the dose (see the dotted line in Figure 3.9). Because more insulin is required between 4:00 A.M. to 10:00 A.M. to keep a person normal while sleeping or waking up (perhaps this increased insulin requirement is due to the lack of exercise plus the rising anti-insulin wake-up hormones), more Ultralente is needed at the evening meal. If the Ultralente is given at 6:00 P.M., its onset is at 10:00 P.M. and it will last until noon the following day (see Figure 3.10). To cover the "hole" between noon and 10:00 P.M., an injection of Ultralente is given at 8:00 A.M. This dose needs to be significantly less than the 6:00 P.M. dose, for three reasons. First, since Ultralente lasts eighteen hours, there will be a "collision" at 10:00 P.M. when the 6:00 P.M. dose of Ultralente starts to work. Second, since Regular insulin is injected around meals, the leftover between-meal Regular adds to the undercurrent of Ultralente. Third, exercise during the day decreases the insulin requirement relative to the lack of exercise at

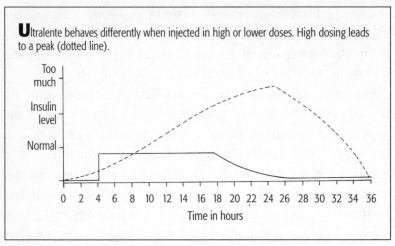

Figure 3.9 Ultralente Injected in High Doses

night (see Figure 3.11). Finally, the newer human Ultralente insulins tend to reach their peak sooner than animal derived Ultralentes. For this reason, it is often necessary to give the evening dose later (9 P.M. to midnight) to "fix the fasting."

As with the NPH insulins, the marriage of Ultralente and Regular is calculated on the basis of body weight. However, since the Ultralente is broken down at the injection site to a greater extent than the NPH family, the total insulin dose for 24 hours is calculated as 0.7 units per kilogram body weight in 24 hours. This dose is actually calculated in two parts because of the need to "gimmick" up the amount of Ultralente to make it as strong as the NPH in our previous example. Thus the Ultralente is calculated as 0.4 units per kilogram of weight, and the Regular is calculated separately as 0.3 units per kilogram. This Regular dose is the total insulin needed to cover all the meals and snacks necessary to maintain the present body weight.

If the patient in our earlier example, Ann, were on this system, her insulin requirements would total 42 units. This total

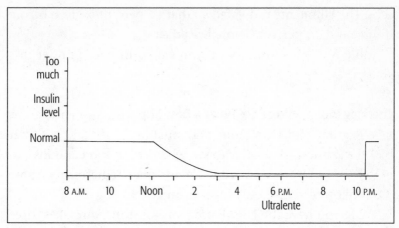

Figure 3.10 Overnight Profile of Low Dose Ultralente

dose is composed of 0.4 units × 60 kilograms = 24 units of Ultralente and 0.3 units × 60 kilograms = 18 units of Regular. The breakfast insulin needs are a bit higher (40 percent of meal needs) because in the morning you are more resistant to insulin. Lunch is 30 percent of meal needs, and dinner is also 30 per-

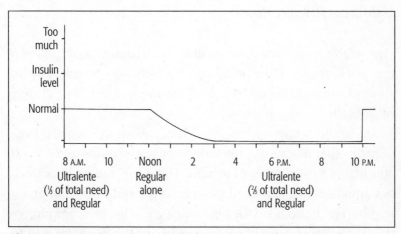

Figure 3.11 Matching Low Dose Ultralente (2 injections) with Regular to Mimic the Normal Pancreas

cent. The Ultralente is divided so that 66 percent is given before dinner and 33 percent before breakfast.

Table 3.7 is a summary of Ann's insulin needs under this system.

Checking Blood Glucose Six Times a Day Suppose Ann chooses to take Regular plus Ultralente. She must make six checks of her blood sugar levels each day to see whether her food and insulin match and to learn what adjustments may be necessary. Table 3.8 is her record of these blood sugar checks:

There you have the Ultralente plan for Ann. Ann takes three injections a day (a mixture of Ultralente and Regular at 8:00 A.M.; Regular at 11:30 A.M.; and Ultralente and Regular at dinnertime).

She's taking a total of 5 doses of insulin daily (2 Ultralente and 3 Regular) and eating three meals. That means she needs six blood glucose readings: three to check the peaks of insulin and three to check the peaks of food. She may also wish to check at 3:00 A.M. to make sure she is not going too low overnight.

Using an Insulin Pump

One of the major advances in diabetes management has been the development of the insulin pump (infusion pump). The insulin pump is designed to deliver insulin in a way that closely mimics the normal situation.

An insulin pump is a small machine, about the size of a pack of cards, that has an insulin syringe or reservoir inside and will automatically give doses of insulin. The pump can be implanted or connected to a needle placed under the skin. Nonimplanted pumps have buttons on the pump that allow for programming of the doses. The pump has tubing with a needle on the end to place under the skin. It is worn on a belt or in a pocket. Im-

TABLE 3.7 A Patient's Insulin Needs

Weight = 60 kilograms
Insulin units = 42 = (0.4 × 60 kilograms = 24 units Ultralente) + (0.3 × 60 kilograms = 18 units Regular)

Breakfast

Breakfast injection. Mixture of Ultralente and Regular: 33% of 24 units of Ultralente = 8 units of Ultralente; 40% of 18 units of Regular = 7.2, round to 7 units of Regular. The scale for Regular still goes up and down by 2 units, as follows:

Prebreakfast Blood Sugar Level	Regular Insulin
Under 70	5 units
70–100	7
100–140	9
Over 140	11

Lunch

Lunch injection. Regular insulin only: 30% of 18 units = 5.4 units of Regular. Now Ann has a choice. If she rounds down to 5 units to cover lunch, she can only eat 5 units' worth of food. Since 5.4 units covers a meal that will maintain Ann's body weight over time, Ann will lose weight. If she rounds up to 6 units, she needs to eat 6 units' worth of food. Over time she will gain weight. As a friend, let's suggest that Ann eats only 5 units at lunch. By the way, Ann is only five foot two. The scale for Regular is as follows:

Prelunch Blood Sugar Level	Regular Insulin
Under 70	3 units
70–100	5
100–140	9
Over 140	9

Dinner

Dinner injection. Ultralente and Regular together in the same syringe: 66% of 24 units of Ultralente = 16 units Ultralente; 30% of 18 units Regular = 5.4 units of Regular. Here, too, Ann must round off the figure. Perhaps since she had a light lunch she can splurge on a 6-unit dinner. The scale for the dinner thus becomes:

Predinner Blood Sugar Level	Regular Insulin
Under 70	4 units
70–100	6
100–140	8
Over 140	10

Each injection of Regular must be injected in enough time before the meal to allow absorption into the bloodstream. The suggestion given in Table 3.2, in which one makes serial blood sugar determinations after an injection to see when the blood sugar has fallen 15 points, can also be used with this system.

planted pumps are available but are considered experimental at the moment.

Earning the Pump Jill earned her pump. Three months ago she was referred for insulin pump therapy. She had erratic glucose control on two injections of insulin a day, although she monitored her blood glucose twice a day.

In order to qualify for insulin pump therapy, Jill had to prove that she was willing to take on the required responsibility. Pump therapy can only be safely prescribed if patients are willing to monitor their blood glucose four to six times a day.

To qualify for her pump, Jill was placed on four injections a day consisting of a combination of NPH before breakfast and bed with three injections of Regular, one before each meal. She was asked to monitor her blood glucose six to eight times a day: before and one hour after each meal, before bed, and at 3:00 A.M. Jill quickly achieved excellent glucose control. Eight weeks later her initial HbA_{1c} of 10 percent had fallen to 6.5 percent. Jill had proved that she was willing to work and could manage intensive insulin therapy if her pump should fail. She was therefore ready for her pump.

Beginning Insulin Prescriptions for the Pump: Calculation of the Basal Infusion Rates Most people will require at least three infusion rates: midnight to 4:00 A.M.; 4:00 A.M. to 10:00 A.M.; and 10:00 A.M. to midnight. The lowest basal dose is usually midnight to 4:00 A.M., concomitant with the nadir of the anti-insulin hormones cortisol and growth hormone. During the early morning hours, 4:00 A.M. to 10:00 A.M., cortisol and growth hormone rise; after 10:00 A.M. they start to fall again. The basal insulin requirement is based on body weight. When anti-insulin hormone levels increase (i.e., with the body's daily cycles, the menstrual cycle, pregnancy, puberty, steroid therapy, etc.), the basal insulin requirement will

TABLE 3.8 Insulin to Carbohydrate Ratio

Blood Glucose	Units*
<70	= 5 (2 units less than calculated)
71–100	= 7 (calculated)
101–140	= 9 (2 units more than calculated)
>141	= 11 (4 units more than calculated)

*Insulin per 70 grams of carbohydrate

rise. Stress, whether illness or emotional state, will also cause the basal requirement to rise. The basal requirement will decrease if exercise in the form of a cardiovascular workout is superimposed on the day's schedule. Thus, although three basal requirements are assumed, the 10:00 A.M. to midnight period may need to be further subdivided.

The best place to begin is to start with one uniform basal infusion calculated to be 0.3 unit per kilogram (kg) per 24 hours for a person who is neither insulin resistant nor sensitive. For an 80-kg (177-pound) person, this turns out to be 24 units per 24 hours, or 1.0 unit per hour. Generally, it is best to initiate pump therapy after 4:00 P.M. because most patients will have taken their morning intermediate insulin doses, which begin to wane about 4:00 P.M.

These basal insulin doses are adjusted systematically. The goal is to go to bed with a blood glucose of 100–150 mg/dl. Ideally, a perfect basal insulin infusion rate does not require snacks to prevent subsequent hypoglycemia. Therefore, a crucial question is what basal will allow a person to go to bed with a normal blood glucose and make it to 4:00 A.M. without drifting up or down. On the initial basal (in our 80-kg person, it is 1.0 unit per hour), the blood glucose is measured at 4:00 A.M. The following night's midnight to 4:00 A.M. basal is adjusted downward by 0.1 unit per hour if the blood glucose is less than 80, and adjusted upward by 0.1 unit per hour if the 4:00 A.M. basal is greater than 110. Once the 4:00 A.M. blood glucose is near a target value of 100, then the 4:00 A.M. to 10:00 A.M. basal is adjusted.

Most people find that their blood glucose drifts up after 4:00 A.M. Therefore, blood glucose should be measured on awakening (8:00 A.M.). If each unit of insulin prevents a blood glucose rise of about 25 mg/dl, and if the 4:00 A.M. blood glucose was 100 mg/dl and the 8:00 A.M. was 200 mg/dl, then 4 extra units of insulin are needed over these four hours, or an additional 1.0 unit per hour (Figure 3.12). In this case, the 1.0 unit per hour needs to be raised to 2.0 units per hour. This higher basal rate usually needs to be continued until 10:00 A.M. The 10:00 A.M.

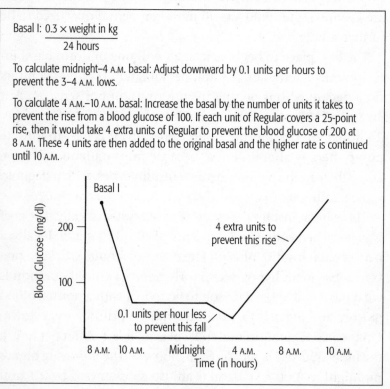

Figure 3.12 Adjusting the Basal Infusion Rate

to midnight basal should be adjusted similarly as needed, depending on the individual's activity patterns.

Premenstrual hormones, especially progesterone, along with chemicals called cytokines and chemokines, tend to potentiate the so-called dawn phenomenon (rise in morning blood sugar). Therefore, menstruating women may find that during the last five days of their cycle, they need to increase even further their 4:00 A.M. to 10:00 A.M. basal infusion rate.

Scheduled Exercise. The pump may be disconnected during strenuous exercise if desired. Depending upon their fitness level, some people may be able to disconnect the pump without requiring a disconnect bolus ("quick" dose) to cover the time off the pump. Until an optimum fitness level is achieved, however, most people need a disconnect bolus equal to approximately one-half the hourly rate, assuming one hour off the pump. Thus, if our 80 kg woman (who requires 1.0 unit per hour from 10:00 A.M. to midnight) wants to exercise from 2:00 to 3:00 P.M., she should bolus 0.5 unit at 2:00 P.M., disconnect the pump until 3:00 P.M., and then reconnect with the original rate of 1.0 unit per hour.

Once our 80 kg woman becomes fit, she will require less insulin and may not need a disconnect bolus. Furthermore, her basal requirement may decrease around the clock. The exercise session will utilize sufficient glucose to keep the patient normal without extra insulin. This same patient may need a reconnect bolus to counteract a phenomenon of postexercise hyperglycemia once the exercising muscles stop utilizing glucose substrate. Since exercise-related insulin doses require meticulous calculations of the basal, based on the blood glucose levels before, during, and after exercise, an attempt at deriving an exercise basal infusion rate should only be made if the patient's basals have been stabilized prior to the addition of the confounding variables associated with exercise.

Meal-Related Insulin Doses: The Bolus If the basal infusion rate is perfectly calculated, then glucose levels will be perfect during fasting, and a meal-related bolus will be required each time the patient eats. A "perfect basal" means that there is no extra insulin around to cover even a snack. A rule of thumb is that each unit of Regular insulin covers 10 grams of carbohydrate for lunch and dinner, but 1.5 units of Regular insulin is required for 10 grams of carbohydrate at breakfast. Although "gluconeogenic amino acids" in protein along with fat may in part eventually convert to glucose in the body, the after-meal blood glucose peak is primarily dependent on the carbohydrate content of the meal. Thus, it is helpful to learn to count carbohydrates. The only way to "learn the carbos" is to look up foods in a reference book. We use Barbara Kraus's *Calories and Carbohydrates*, published by Signet, which lists over 8,000 brand names and basic foods.

For a weight maintenance diet, most women require 22 to 25 calories per kilogram of weight per day, depending on their exercise level. Most men require 25 to 35 calories per kilogram. Thus, our 80-kg woman who does not exercise needs 1,760 calories a day to maintain her weight. Her "carbohydrate quota" is calculated to be 40 percent of her calories. Each gram of carbohydrate is equivalent to about 4 calories. Her "carbo quota" (allowance of grams of carbohydrate per day) is determined based on the following formula:

$$\frac{80 \text{ kg} \times 22 \text{ calories} \times 40\%}{4} = \text{grams of carbo} = \text{quota per 24 hours}$$

Thus, $1,760 \times 0.1 = 176$ grams of carbo = quota per 24 hours.

The distribution of carbohydrates consumed throughout the day will be according to individual preference, but most people will note that they tolerate very little carbohydrate before 10:00 A.M., essentially during the time their "dawn phenomenon" with its counter-insulin hormone surge is at its peak. In fact, as noted

TABLE 3.9 Insulin to Carbohydrate Ratio

Blood Glucose	Units*
<70 = 5 (2 units less than calculated)
71–100 = 7 (calculated)
101–140 = 9 (2 units more than calculated)
>141 = 11 (4 units more than calculated)

*Insulin per 70 grams of carbohydrate

above, eating carbohydrates between 4:00 A.M. and 10:00 A.M. requires 1.5 units of Regular insulin per 10 grams of carbohydrate. After 10:00 A.M., the insulin-to-carbo ratio is usually 1 unit per 10 grams. The patient should try out these ratios and adjust them based on the blood glucose level one hour after a meal.

Let's say, for example, that a person wants to eat 70 grams of carbo for a 1:00 P.M. lunch. At the rate of 1 unit per 10 grams of carbo, this would call for 7 units of Regular insulin. This is the right amount of insulin to cover the meal plan alone, but the dose also needs adjusting based on the premeal blood glucose level (see Table 3.9).

Then let's say that the blood glucose one hour after the meal was 225. If the goal is to be no higher than 150 one hour after the meal, and if each unit of insulin prevents a 25-point rise, 3 more units (or 10 units total) are needed to cover the 70 grams of carbohydrate. This person's ratio is thus 10 units of insulin for 70 grams of carbohydrate, or 1 unit of insulin for 7 grams of carbohydrate.

Figure 3.13 shows the daily adjustment chart insulin-pump patients keep while their ratios are being derived. At the beginning, it is easier if only fixed amounts of carbohydrate are eaten. Once the ratios are derived, the meal plan may become much more flexible.

Date						
Basal Rates Midnight–4 A.M.						
4 A.M.–10 A.M.						
10 A.M.–Midnight						
Other Basals						
Meal-related Boluses Breakfast						
BS < 70						
71–100						
101–140						
> 141						
Lunch						
BS < 70						
71–100						
101–140						
> 141						
Dinner						
BS < 70						
71–100						
101–140						
> 141						

Figure 3.13 Flow Sheet for Insulin Pump Therapy

The Lag Time It is easy to create "brittle" (unstable) diabetes: all you need to do is eat too soon after you "bolus" the premeal insulin dose. The simple sugars in the food will reach the bloodstream in fifteen minutes. The subcutaneously injected insulin will not even begin to reach the bloodstream for at least thirty to forty-five minutes, and will not peak for two to three hours. The only way to have the food and the insulin meet the bloodstream at the same moment is to "bolus" the premeal dose about thirty to forty-five minutes before eating. Rates of absorption also varies with needle site placement, scarring of the skin, and inflammation. Different insulin types also have different lag times. Thus as with insulin injections, it is important to determine your own personal lag time for your pumped insulin. A warning about lag times: Do not anticipate food in a restaurant by bolusing your insulin before you see your food. What happens more often than not is that the food will not arrive and you will have to eat the sugar dish to avoid hypoglycemia—a waste of a dining out experience!

Diligence Is Required In summary, once a patient "earns" the pump, then a systematic approach to the calculation and adjustment of the insulin doses should be implemented. As a safety measure, when starting pump therapy, at least eight blood glucose checks need to be performed: before and one hour after each meal, before bed, and at 3:00 to 4:00 A.M. Only when stable sugars are established can the frequency of monitoring be decreased. Special situations that need increased monitoring include the premenstrual period, infection, stress, and exercise. Although more flexible than multiple injections, the pump requires diligent effort to keep the system safe and functioning well.

With practice, you will be able to develop great skills in anticipating calories and adjusting insulin—even without the need to bracket the meal with blood glucose measurements. However, don't abandon them completely, for changes in blood glucose levels can occur without your sensing them.

Whatever your system, the key is to maintain normal blood glucose throughout the day. There is no "right" or "wrong" system—only one that works for you.

More About Insulin

There are a few other points that you should know about insulin in addition to its action and duration. Insulin comes in varying strengths. We recommend U-100 to our diabetic patients because it is easier to use and calibrate. But whatever strength insulin you use, it should be consistent with your syringe type. Syringes are calibrated to hold one milliliter (1 ml) or cubic centimeter (1 cc) of insulin. This volume remains constant, regardless of the unit of insulin specified. Because small children may require doses of ½ unit or less, it is sometimes helpful to dilute insulin. Special dilution solutions are available for this purpose.

When you divide your injections into split doses and combinations of insulins, it is especially important to accurately measure the exact amounts since half a unit may make a large difference in your blood glucose once control is achieved. Low-dose syringes can be most helpful for this purpose. These syringes have large calibration scales and can be read to within half a unit. You should be careful, too, to mix insulin without contaminating one bottle of insulin with another. The proper method of mixing insulins is illustrated in Figure 3.14. Basically it requires that you inject an appropriate amount of air into each bottle and then withdraw the insulin in sequence to avoid cross-contamination between bottles.

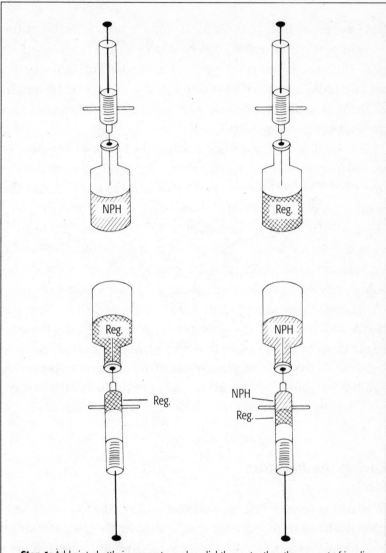

Step 1: Add air to bottle in amount equal or slightly greater than the amount of insulin needed so there is no suction to bottle.

Step 2: Withdraw insulin from each bottle in the amount needed, being careful not to contaminate one insulin bottle with insulin from the other. Put Regular into syringe first, then NPH.

Figure 3.14 Mixing Insulin

Pen Devices A clever and useful invention now available is the insulin pen. The insulin pen is a device similar to a fountain pen, with a cartridge full of insulin instead of ink in the barrel and a needle instead of a writing tip. The dose is set by a twist of the dial, and a depression of the plunger delivers the exact amount of insulin required.

The insulin pen has several advantages. It provides a discrete way to take insulin. The stigma of carrying needles and syringes is not attached to a "fountain pen." It's handy as well, because the insulin, needle, and syringe all come ready to use. A shopping bag of supplies is no longer necessary. With smaller needles, pen devices may be less painful than conventional injection. The needle never has to go through a rubber stopper to draw up insulin; the insulin is pushed through the needle on the end opposite to the needle. Therefore, the needle tip tends to stay sharper. The sharper the needle, the less it hurts. Using the pen is also more accurate than trying to draw up insulin to a line on a syringe and then trying to snap out all the bubbles. Finally, use of the pen and longer acting insulins facilitates a way to more easily mimic the basal-bolus approach to insulin delivery that makes the pump so attractive.

Giving the Injection

In addition to your insulin, you should have the following supplies on hand to prepare for your injection: the proper syringe and needle, alcohol, and cotton. Swabbing the injection area with alcohol will clean the site, but allow the alcohol to dry to take some of the sting out of the procedure.

In any case, you should quickly insert the needle under the skin and then attempt to withdraw the plunger a bit to see if you have penetrated a blood vessel. If blood does appear, withdraw the syringe and start all over again. If no blood appears, complete the injection. After total injection, withdraw the needle and replace the needle cap, then dispose of the syringe and needle properly.

If you inadvertently inject into a vein, the insulin will peak within twenty to forty-five minutes and you might find yourself severely hypoglycemic. This is a rare occurrence but can be quite frightening. If you think you have administered insulin into a vein, you should test your blood sugar every fifteen minutes to make sure your glucose levels are not dropping too rapidly. You may also want to take glucagon, a hormone that raises glucose and is described later on in the chapter.

Rotating injection sites will help to avoid problems of *lipodystrophy*, scarring or fatty changes in the fat tissue under the skin which occur from injecting extensively in one area. This can lead to loss of subcutaneous fat or sometimes actual accumulation of fat in one area with a result that can be unsightly and also lead to erratic insulin absorption. Site rotation is especially helpful if split dosages are used. Figure 3.15 indicates the many sites from which you have to choose. Once you select one, clean the area thoroughly before inserting the needle. The side of the needle is beveled to provide a sharp cutting edge for easier penetration of the skin. In general, this beveled side should be pointed up during injection.

If you use an insulin pump, you may wish to "disconnect" at times and use standard insulin injection techniques. A good example would be during times you are at the beach or swimming. Since pump systems generally use regular insulin in a specific dilution, you can mimic your pump action by injecting the appropriate amount hourly or every two or three hours, and before eating. This may be done by injecting Regular insulin either through the pump tubing or by subcutaneous injection or an insulin pen. If you use the pump tubing, remember that some insulin remains in the tube and will not be available to the body.

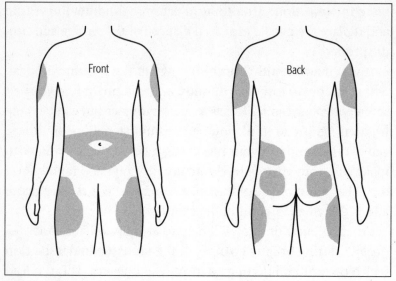

Figure 3.15 Site of Insulin Injections

If you wish to use the pump tubing, discuss it first with your physician.

Your Changing Needs

It is important to understand that when insulin requirements change, there is generally a reason for it. Pregnant diabetic women, for example, require increasingly more insulin with each month of pregnancy than they did before they became pregnant. People who are under stress require more insulin whether the stress is caused by emotion or infection. Children reaching puberty or having a growth spurt require increased insulin, sometimes to the point of doubling their requirements in a relatively short time primarily in the overnight dose. These increases are natural, but if it is not clear to you why your insulin needs are so much greater at a certain time, you should see your physician to help find the cause. At any rate, keep tabs on your blood glucose levels, and you can handle interim problems until you see your physician. You are in charge of the situation and need no longer be afraid when your body is doing something "funny." You now have the skills to cope with it, but you may need help in learning exactly what is going on.

Your insulin requirements may also increase when your pancreas is no longer able to produce as much insulin as it once did. The better you are at helping your pancreas early, the longer it may keep working with you even if at only a partial level of activity. It is much easier to control your diabetes if your pancreas is helping. For this reason, it is important to keep your blood glucose between 50 and 150 mg/dl as best you can. You can tell if your pancreas is working by calculating how much insulin you take. A person with no pancreatic function requires about 0.6 unit of insulin per kilogram of body weight. If you weigh 110 pounds (50 kg), you need about 30 units a day to maintain normal blood glucose levels. If you are using less than that and keeping in the normal glucose range with 20 units of insulin, your pancreas must be supplying the other 10. You can also tell if you are insulin resistant by seeing if your requirements are greater than 0.6 unit of insulin per kg/body weight.

Certainly with insulin-dependent diabetes, the sooner you begin insulin therapy, and the better you control your blood glucose, the longer the pancreas may be able to produce insulin and help to do the job it once did by itself. We have known patients who required only a couple of units of insulin a day and yet kept their pancreas working for them for periods up to twenty years. Eventually the pancreas will tire and your insulin requirements will increase, but it is important to help it work for you as long as it can.

GLUCAGON AND FAST-ACTING SUGAR SOURCES

Diabetic patients should also have another injectable preparation on hand—glucagon. This hormone counteracts insulin and will raise the blood glucose when it is too low. It is injected like insulin under the skin. Glucagon is supplied in a vial that contains the hormone plus liquid to dilute the preparation. If hypoglycemia does occur and is such that the diabetic person cannot respond with fast-acting sugar, a friend or relative should be prepared to administer glucagon. This rarely happens, but it is best to be prepared.

You can calibrate glucagon like insulin. Ten to 20 units on your insulin syringe (this equals 0.10 to 0.15 mg of glucagon; glucagon comes in "one-unit vials," which contain 1 mg) will raise the blood glucose by about 30 mg/dl in fifteen to thirty minutes in an adult. For example, if you awaken and take your insulin and then you find you are ill and vomiting, all you have to do is measure your blood glucose and inject enough glucagon to raise your blood glucose to about 100 mg/dl. The glucagon effect lasts about three hours.

Here is where your daily diary is so important. You will have noted in it when you became hypoglycemic and at what blood glucose levels you started to feel different. You will also have noted that your blood glucose rises after you eat and at a predictable amount after you eat certain foods. Now you can learn to calculate exactly how much specific foods raise your blood glucose, a technique that will help you to correct a hypoglycemic episode early without leaping into a vicious cycle of blood glucose swings winding up in hyperglycemia.

You can, of course, select a fast-acting, or simple sugar (simple syrup, candy, etc.) to respond to hypoglycemic episodes. A candy that we have found particularly helpful is called Honee, made in Italy by G.B. Ambroselli and available in the United States. It has a liquid honey core for a fast sugar source, and it does not melt in hot weather. One piece raises the blood glucose level of a person weighing 50 kg by about 20 mg/dl. Therefore, four of these candies are usually sufficient to correct any hypoglycemic episode until you can eat your scheduled meal or snack. There are also many commercially available glucose sources especially for persons with diabetes.

No matter what you use as a fast-acting sugar source, it will help you to know just how much it raises your blood glucose level. Half a glass of orange juice, for instance, usually produces a rise of about 100 mg/dl, but this will vary from one individual to another depending on weight.

To calibrate how your particular blood glucose reacts to a simple sugar, wait until your level is below 120 mg/dl on the glucose meter, and then take your sugar source. Fifteen minutes to one-half hour later, measure your blood glucose and record the results in your diary. Once you have done this with several portable foods, you are prepared to cope with any hypoglycemic episode in an appropriate manner.

You are now ready to experiment with other foods to determine how soon they peak in your bloodstream. Since this varies from one person to another, let your glucose meter be your guide. In general, simple sugars peak in about fifteen to thirty minutes, which is why they are used to combat hypoglycemia. Complex sugars peak anywhere from thirty minutes to an hour, fats and starches in about one to one-and-a-half hours after a meal, and proteins in approximately three hours.

The problem with simple sugars is that they not only peak quickly but they also fall off quickly in terms of blood glucose. Therefore, a useful protocol to follow for low glucose is this: If you feel hypoglycemic, document it. Your first sign may be tingling around the mouth. If your glucose is below 70 mg/dl, drink a glass (240 cc or 150 calories) of whole milk and record your glucose in fifteen minutes. Repeat this if necessary. If this does not work, then have a third glass of milk plus one slice of bread. This last step is hardly ever necessary. Because milk is a complex food (carbohydrate, fat, and protein), it will tend to tide you over better than simple-sugar-type foods.

The amount you eat also makes a difference in terms of when the food peaks as glucose in your bloodstream. The greater the load, the longer it will take your stomach to absorb all the food. If you eat a huge meal just before you go to sleep, you may not realize its maximum effect until you awaken in the morning (known in the United States as the Thanksgiving effect).

Once you know when certain foods peak in your bloodstream, you are much freer to substitute foods that have the same effect on your blood glucose level. You also have a handy guideline to calibrate your insulin dosage to correspond to the time when your food peaks. This is essentially the key to optimum control—to design your insulin peaks to coincide with the way your food is absorbed. It can become quite easy, but it demands consistency in what you eat, when you take your insulin, and when you exercise. Furthermore, everything should be recorded at first in your daily diary. In time, you will rely less on reacting to problems and more on anticipating and avoiding them.

Now that you have learned to measure your own blood glucose and combine this procedure with optimum therapy, it is time to learn about how your particular system responds in terms of blood glucose swings and in relation to different foods. After that, we shall discuss reasonable meal planning and selecting your food types intelligently so that you can begin to fine-tune your diabetes control.

4

Blood Glucose Swings and Your Mood

When Ralph was discharged from the Army ten years ago, his physical examination indicated a high blood glucose level. He was advised to consult a physician in civilian life but neglected to do so. Now he was having difficulty walking and maintaining his balance and was very depressed. His toes dropped down, and he had to keep his feet farther apart and lift them higher to avoid tripping. Finally, he went to the doctor and discovered that his blood glucose level was almost 300 mg/dl and his hemoglobin A_{1c} was over 10 percent. Ralph had diabetic neuropathy and myopathy (the disease had affected his nerves and muscles to the extent that he was confined to bed). Ralph was told that he would have to control the diabetes before the nerves could even begin to heal. He was also told that with optimum therapy, the situation might get better. Ralph's hope of improvement motivated him to intensify his treatment program.

The prediction proved correct. After three months of normal glycemia, he gradually improved, first in a wheelchair, then with a walker, and finally with braces. Eighteen months later, he no longer requires braces and is walking well. His strength is *returning and exercises have helped to tone his muscles. The pains which kept him awake at night are gone, and he is in better physical condition than he has been for a long time. His depression also lifted as his HbA$_{1c}$ levels approached the normal range.*

R alph's case proves that the goal of optimum control is well worth any effort. By learning to measure your own blood glucose and adjust your insulin dosage, you are on the way to achieving this goal. This does not mean you will not have problems. You may still be plagued by blood glucose swings as foods and moods affect your glucose levels more than you had realized. Your aim is to keep your blood glucose between 50 and 150 mg/dl, and the more you learn about yourself and how your system reacts to sudden changes, the closer you will come to this ideal.

With food, you can learn to anticipate elevations and calibrate your insulin accordingly. Changes brought on by mood and/or stress, however, are more difficult to anticipate, but in time you can learn to handle even these in a predictable manner.

Blood glucose affects mood in at least two ways, and of course mood affects your blood glucose. Getting upset or angry may lead to an elevation in blood glucose of over 200 mg/dl. Watch out, though, because this may be followed by an equally large drop. Stress seems to lead to alternating high and low blood glucose levels. The temptation is to give a little extra insulin in response to the high blood glucose level following stressful situations. This response tends to make the subsequent drop in glucose worse and lead to a severe hypoglycemic reaction as well, and the roller coaster of highs and lows begins. A better approach is to try to come to terms with the stress itself and be gentle in responding with either insulin or food. It is better to wait until the next scheduled dose of insulin and respond at that time with the adjustment than to panic and inject extra insulin at the moment and risk making the situation worse.

There are certain persons who have an abnormal stress response which they cannot turn off. In certain types of stressful situations, these individuals continue to elevate their blood glucose until they end up in ketoacidosis (high acid and fat breakdown products called ketones in the blood) despite the fact that they are increasing the insulin dose. The problem in this case is not with insulin delivery but with the person's response to stress. The key to treatment is to get at the cause of the stress. Most of the patients with this problem tend to be teenagers who are often caught in family conflicts. Family therapy for about nine months has been shown to help these diabetic persons and their families avoid the frequent hospitalizations and bouts of hyperglycemia by coping better with the stress of their lives.

Everyone knows that low blood glucose can affect mood in dramatic ways. However, as you become more accustomed to having normal blood glucose levels, the changes in mood during hypoglycemia become more subtle. It is important to be sensitive to even the slightest change in mood. Family members should be encouraged to suggest that the person with diabetes check blood glucose when there is any question of an unusual although subtle mood change.

Research has shown that high blood glucose over time also has an impact on mood. Specifically, persons with high glycosylated hemoglobin values have been shown to be more depressed than those with values closer to normal. The depression scores tend to correct as blood glucose values come down toward normal as measured by hemoglobin A_{1c} values.

A number of factors improve as glucose control as reflected by hemoglobin A_{1c} improves. Feelings of depression lift. You have more energy. That "weight" of inner pain that you had been carrying for so long and could not explain begins to go away.

It is also interesting to note that as people begin to take better care of themselves and control their blood glucose, excessive worrying about health in general appears to decrease. Thus, the once-hypochondriac becomes a health advocate and replaces useless worries about a multitude of potential problems with useful activities directed at the real problem of controlling blood glucose.

Children with high blood glucose levels may become quite different little people once their blood sugar levels are lower. The diabetic child who has been withdrawn, incommunicative, sullen, and appeared almost retarded, can return to being a happy, bouncy child with the help of normal blood glucose levels.

You can see that the work involved in maintaining near-normal blood glucose levels pays off in several ways, including the fact that you will probably feel better. The hopeless and helpless feelings that you may have had regarding life and diabetes may have been due in part merely to the fact that your blood sugar has been too high for a while. This can be fixed, and you should have hope that in the not too distant future you will begin to feel better in many ways.

This is not to say that all depression in persons with diabetes is related to blood glucose. Depression is common and if symptoms do not improve with improved glucose levels, further professional help and medication may be warranted. It is difficult to care for oneself if one is depressed. Therefore, it is sometimes useful to treat the depression first so that the person with diabetes has the renewed energy to care for him or herself.

5

Food and Meal Planning

Mary has had diabetes since age ten. Now in her early thirties, she was often depressed and experienced severe pain in her hands and legs. When she finally saw her doctor, her hemoglobin A_{1C} was 17 percent. Mary's problem was food—or rather too much food. She craved it constantly. When she couldn't sleep at night, she ate. When she was up during the day, she ate. Her life was one continuous refrigerator raid. With her doctor's help, Mary learned to measure her blood glucose levels and to distribute her insulin injections. But her hemoglobin A_{1C} remained at 9 percent because Mary still went on food binges. Her blood glucose would go as high as 400 mg/dl at these times, but she was afraid to use enough insulin to bring it down because of the possibility of shock. Since she couldn't or wouldn't control her food intake, Mary was hospitalized to stabilize her blood glucose. But as soon as she was discharged, she was off and running to the refrigerator, and the same pattern repeated itself. Finally, Mary came to grips with her problem and went to a nutrition consultant. The dietitian worked with Mary's physician to alter her eating habits and, in time, normalize her hemoglobin A_{1c}. Today Mary is active in a job she likes and maintains good dietary habits.

Mary's food problem may be extreme, but she is certainly not alone in her eating habits. Americans are bombarded on all sides by ads and commercials urging us to eat simple sugars and junk foods. We not only consume too many calories, we eat the wrong kind of calories. This is not good for anyone—but it can be disastrous for the person with diabetes.

The key to good meal planning is to know the optimum number of calories for your body weight and distribute those calorie in a rational way throughout the day. This can be done by counting calories, counting carbohydrates, or by using the exchange system. Food should be distributed fairly evenly during the day. Snacks may be planned throughout the day to give your

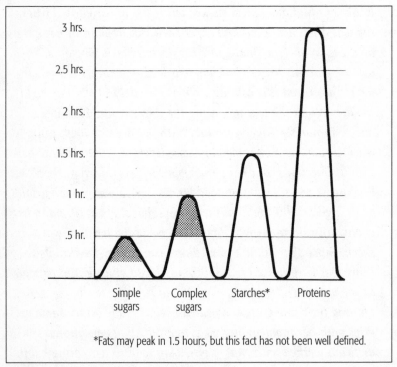

*Fats may peak in 1.5 hours, but this fact has not been well defined.

Figure 5.1 Peak Absorption Time of Foods

body a constant fuel supply to go with your insulin dosage. In a previous chapter, you learned how to determine when your insulin peaks. From this you can calculate your calorie needs and know how best to distribute them to avoid erratic blood glucose swings and maintain constant glucose levels.

Once you have mastered the proper use of food, your battle with diabetes is 90 percent over. Glucose measurements will help you do this. You have already begun to measure the peak for different types of foods and have found that simple carbohydrates, or sugars, peak at about fifteen to thirty minutes. Complex carbohydrates take anywhere from thirty minutes to an hour, fats and starches peak in approximately ninety minutes, and proteins take the longest to convert to blood sugar—about three hours (see Figure 5.1). When you plan your meals, then, you should be aware of these peaks and compare them with when your insulin peaks. A mixed meal peaks in about one hour.

COUNTING CALORIES

The amount of food needed varies for each individual, depending on body composition, weight, and level of activity. In general, moderately active adults require an average of 25 calories per kilogram of weight per day. For example, if you weigh 50 kg (110 pounds), you need about 1,250 calories per day to maintain your present body weight. However, you should not put yourself into a mathematical box. The important thing, especially for children, is not to feel hungry and to maintain or gain weight at a normal level.

People who have high blood glucose levels also are "hyperphagic" (they eat more). Therefore, when you normalize your blood glucose levels, not only will you eat less, but you also will be less hungry, since the calories you do eat will be utilized and not wasted. The first week of establishing more normal blood glucose levels is the most difficult since the "binge cravings" will persist for about that long.

There is still some controversy as to what constitutes the best diet for diabetic patients. Books on diet and diet fads abound for diabetic and nondiabetic persons alike, and many are touted with missionary zeal. The diabetic person should follow reasonable meal planning patterns, which are best for everyone. This means avoiding simple sugars, which, if nothing else, can ruin your teeth. It also means being especially aware of the peak absorption times of different foods in your bloodstream and the consequences of excess weight gain. With your glucose measurements, you can decide what is the best meal plan for you and tailor a diet to meet your specific needs. In time, you will become so expert in proper meal planning, you may encourage your nondiabetic friends to learn the principles of good nutrition.

Remember, there is no magic diet that fits everyone all the time. You need to find the nutrition plan that is best for you and tailor it to fit your needs. Calories and carbohydrates generally receive the most attention in meal planning. However, you also need to be aware of how your diet is impacting on other health issues as well. Do you need to have a special diet that helps you achieve better blood pressure levels? Do you have high uric acid levels and therefore need to modify your diet for that reason? Are your blood lipid levels abnormal and therefore do you need to have a diet that helps you lower your cholesterol and triglycerides? For persons with diabetes, the first step is to fix glucose levels because this will often help fix other problems such as lipids and blood pressure. For many individuals, fixing the glucose levels is a first step on the way to improved health through an increasingly improved diet. The key with diet, as with medications is to try an improvement, see if it works, and then improve it further.

After calculating your total calories, you are ready to plan their distribution. You can convert the total calories into appropriate food exchanges with the aid of convenient tables available from insulin manufacturers, the American Diabetes Association, Juvenile Diabetes Foundation, American Dietetic Association, and other sources in your area.

Once you have assessed your caloric requirements and eliminated many simple sugars, you need to distribute your calories in a way that helps you normalize your blood glucose. Remember, the goal is to keep your blood glucose in the normal range, not to adhere to some rigid diet formula.

COUNTING CARBOHYDRATES

The easiest way to match insulin to calories is to learn the carbohydrate content of foods. With this skill you can predict how much Regular it will take for you to cover a given meal. Remember, it takes more insulin to cover a certain amount of carbohydrate at breakfast or between 4:00 and 10:00 A.M. than it does throughout the rest of the day. Most persons need about 1.5 units of insulin for every 10 grams of carbohydrate ingested in the morning, but only about 1 unit of insulin for every 10 grams of carbohydrate in the afternoon and evening. Once this ratio is calculated for you, it becomes relatively easy to enter a restaurant, look at the plate, and say, "This is a 1,200-calorie 'pig out' with about 110 grams of carbohydrate. I'm going to eat the whole thing and therefore I need 11 units of insulin." This type of calculation becomes easy with practice but is difficult at first, so you may want to work with a nutritionist for a few sessions until you begin to master it. The advantage of such a system is that you have the freedom to vary the time and amounts of your meals and do not have to feel locked into some rigid diet. It is important that you have an insulin delivery scheme that allows the injection of insulin before each meal in order to make this system work.

Another advantage of the carbohydrate counting method is that you can bank your calories and insulin. This means that if you are matching insulin to food correctly, you have a check on how much you are eating and can avoid excess weight gain merely by limiting the amount of insulin you are going to use to cover food during a given twenty-four-hour period. A number of centers are now developing computer programs to help you calculate calories and carbohydrates, and match insulin to food.

BALANCING MEALS

Most people eat about 20 percent of their calories as protein, and the balance is divided equally between carbohydrates and fats. However, if you have insulin-dependent diabetes and your pancreas is not functioning at all, you may find that you cannot eat simple sugar in the morning. Our patients with insulin-dependent diabetes tend to eat about 25 percent protein in their diet (and our pregnant diabetic patients eat about 20 percent protein), but the percentages for breakfast are higher. If orange juice raises your blood glucose level 200 mg/dl and peaks in your bloodstream in fifteen to thirty minutes, you would have to get up two hours before breakfast to inject your insulin to cover that peak. Thus you may want to eliminate or postpone your fruit toward the end of breakfast and increase your protein content. You can save fruits for later in the day or calibrate them to go along with exercise.

It is important to have an estimate of how much carbohydrate you eat at each meal. This will let you know if your carbohydrate intake and insulin dose are well matched. Most insulin-dependent individuals find they can eat only about 12 to 20 percent of their total calories for breakfast. The rest of the breakfast calories are made up in snacks or at other meals.

Your meal pattern may vary depending on how much and what types of insulin are used. For example, if you are on three shots of a mixture of intermediate-acting NPH and short-acting Regular insulin a day, you generally will need snacks. However, you can decrease your NPH in the morning and take Regular insulin before lunch. If your lunch is mostly protein, you can figure that your insulin will peak at about the same time as your food and inject Regular insulin just before you eat. On the other hand, if your lunch is low in protein, you will need to inject the insulin up to an hour and a half before you eat, depending on your luncheon menu. In either case, you can determine this by using your glucose measuring system and knowing when your insulin peaks.

The advantage of injecting Regular insulin before lunch is that if you have to skip that meal or have a larger lunch for some reason, you can adjust your Regular insulin accordingly.

The important thing is to be consistent. We are creatures of habit and eat similar meals every day anyway, but this eating pattern is especially important for someone with diabetes. Spacing meals appropriately has several advantages besides making it easier to adjust insulin. Studies have shown that persons who skip meals and eat one large meal at night have poor glucose tolerance, higher cholesterol levels, and a tendency to be overweight. A balanced diet with well-distributed meals is essential to good health, especially for the diabetic for whom it is more important to avoid falling into an obesity-prone meal pattern. You have the skills and the tools to adjust your insulin to almost any type of eating pattern; however, the more healthful your eating habits, the easier it will be to control your diabetes and the better you will feel.

Again, the key to coming to terms with your diabetes is to measure what you are doing. This applies not only to your blood glucose levels as you adjust your insulin and food intake but also to your cholesterol and triglyceride levels. Fats, or lipids, have been implicated in atherosclerosis and vascular disease in persons with diabetes. Usually, as the diabetes is brought under control, the body fats revert to normal. Too much cholesterol in the blood is unhealthful, and eating excess amounts of animal fats can contribute to elevated cholesterol levels.

Still, some fats are necessary in the diet. They account for about 40 percent of the calories we consume and provide certain vitamins needed during the day. Animal or saturated fats are thought to be more harmful than the polyunsaturated fats, which are generally liquid fats of vegetable origin. In the long run, it is better to substitute fats of the polyunsaturated variety in the diet for the saturated fats with high cholesterol content. Even so, our bodies manufacture a certain amount of their own saturated fat, hence further dietary adjustments may be necessary to reduce high blood lipid levels even after diabetes is brought under control.

Another diet controversy involving diabetes is the role of high-carbohydrate, high-fiber diets. With insulin therapy, this debate may not be as crucial as we begin to be more skilled in matching insulin with food. For the type 2 diabetic person, a high-carbohydrate, high-fiber diet has been shown to aid in cutting calories and lowering blood lipid levels so that it is often possible to eliminate insulin entirely. For the type 1 diabetic person, the story is a little trickier. Remember, the goal is to maintain normal blood glucose levels. High-carbohydrate, high-fiber diets are difficult to match with insulin, especially at breakfast, for the reasons mentioned above.

Foods high in fiber include vegetables, fruits, legumes, bran, and oats. The highest fiber content foods are carrots and celery. Cooking will break down the fiber and convert it into easily absorbed carbohydrates. Filling up on high-fiber foods is a way to appease the appetite, keep calorie intake down, and improve normal bowel function. In addition, when you fill up on fiber, you have less room for tempting foods high in fat, calories, and cholesterol. Thus, high-fiber diets are a helpful way to lose weight.

When you are starting to match insulin with food, it is often easier to begin with a 40 percent carbohydrate diet. The reason is that with this percentage, 100 calories are equivalent to 10 grams of carbohydrate. Most of us are better at counting calories than we are at counting carbohydrates, and a diet with a ratio of calories to carbohydrate at 40 percent carbohydrate makes it much easier to learn these systems.

There is no argument, then, against a high-fiber diet for someone with diabetes. The same may be said about following a vegetarian diet. No matter what type of diet is used, the important thing is to measure how it affects your blood glucose and, above all, to be consistent. With your glucose measurements, you can match your insulin to almost any food type, and diabetes control becomes predictable and easy.

A few words should be added for the diabetic person who also has kidney disease. The kidneys clean the bloodstream of the waste products from the food we eat. Protein is necessary as a building block of muscle, but it also produces waste products that can harm an already damaged kidney. Thus, patients with renal disease are usually advised to limit the amount of protein in their diet. Other sources of waste product problems are foods high in the minerals potassium and phosphorus. Tomatoes, peas, and bananas are high in potassium. Dairy products are high in phosphorus. The diet for the diabetic person with kidney failure is also complicated because kidney failure usually produces high blood pressure, and a person with high blood pressure should not eat salt. To come up with a diet that is satisfying, nutritious, and tasty, yet has minimal sugar, salt, dairy products, meat, fat, or fruits takes a very creative dietitian working together with the patient. Thus, a consultation with a dietitian is a must for any diabetic patient with renal disease.

6

Alcohol and Diabetes

Alcohol can be toxic in much the same way that glucose can be, and the two chemicals can "gang up" on a person to make matters much worse. Therefore, you should think twice before drinking if you have diabetes.

We are not insisting that you become a teetotaler. If you are not an alcoholic, you can adjust your insulin to accommodate the occasional drink. All diabetics who drink, however—alcoholic or not—should be aware of what alcohol does to the body.

Many symptoms of alcohol abuse, such as muscle wasting, aches and pains, erratic blood glucose levels, inability to sleep, neuropathy, loss of sex drive, depression, anxiety, and loss of memory or other mental impairment, may be misunderstood as simply conditions often associated with diabetes, when they may in fact result from combining diabetes and alcohol. Alcohol also makes it difficult for the pancreas in some persons to work properly. The purpose of this chapter is to increase your awareness of the problems associated with alcohol in persons

TABLE 6.1 Problems Associated with Alcohol Intake by Persons with Diabetes

Acute: Potentially Life-Threatening

> Hypoglycemia
>
> Ketosis/acidosis

Chronic: Interaction of Alcohol in Diabetic Problems

> Combining with proteins, lipids, and DNA
>
> Changes in food-handling pathways
>
> Nerve and muscle disease (neuropathy/myopathy)
>
> Heart disease/high blood pressure/lipid abnormalities
>
> Brain effects
>
> Liver problems
>
> Cataracts and eye diseases
>
> Bleeding from the kidneys (papillary necrosis)
>
> Vulnerability to infection/immunology problems
>
> Skin changes
>
> Bone changes
>
> Gut disturbances
>
> Complications of pregnancy
>
> Problems with body fat distribution

with diabetes and to describe useful coping strategies that may help avoid tragedy.

WHAT IS WRONG WITH ALCOHOL?

Table 6.1 lists the problems anyone with diabetes mellitus may encounter as a consequence of alcohol ingestion. There are two levels of clinical concern regarding the interaction of glucose and alcohol. The first and primary concern is that the elevation of these two chemicals in excess may lead to acute and life-threatening consequences. The second concern is that the long-term consequences of having elevated amounts of glucose and alcohol worsens the problems associated with diabetes.

Alcohol May Lead to Hypoglycemia and Ketoacidosis

There are two potentially life-threatening consequences of drinking too much for the person with diabetes—in addition to the potential loss of life from an overdose of alcohol or loss of judgment secondary to intoxication. The first and most common is hypoglycemia (low blood sugar); the second is a buildup of acid in the bloodstream (ketosis and acidosis).

Hypoglycemia

There are two phases in the blood glucose response to ingested alcohol. The first is the glucose response to the alcoholic beverage itself and any food that was consumed at the same time. Some alcoholic beverages contain a good deal of carbohydrate or sugar. Always be aware of the carbohydrate content of your drink. A brisk rise in blood glucose after a sugar-laden drink may inspire the taking of additional oral hypoglycemic agents or insulin. This action may be especially hazardous because the second phase of the blood glucose response to alcohol is an inhibition of liver enzymes, helper molecules that mobilize sugar from the liver. The resulting hypoglycemic effect of alcohol may persist from eight to twelve hours after the last drink and may occur following ingestion of amounts consistent with "social drinking." To make matters worse, alcohol also suppresses hormones that help us protect ourselves from low blood sugar (catecholamines, glucagon, and growth hormone).

Ketoacidosis

Chronic alcohol ingestion is sometimes associated with the buildup of certain acids. The occurrence of lactic acidosis appears to require the presence of clinically significant liver disease, and levels of alcohol are usually high in the bloodstream when this problem occurs. The buildup of ketones appears to occur in chronic drinkers who then cease drinking. Cessation of drinking and lack of a proper diet to deplete excess fat stores that have not been mobilized due to the presence of acetate (an acid breakdown product of alcohol) combine to produce excessive fat mobilization and ketosis. To make matters even more complicated, in a person who consumes a fair amount of alcohol, putting a sudden halt to drinking may lead to vomiting, with further worsening of health.

ALCOHOL MAY LEAD TO OR WORSEN THE COMPLICATIONS OF DIABETES

The chronic interaction of alcohol and diabetes is now being studied in detail. Both glucose and acetaldehyde (the first breakdown product of alcohol) are reactive molecules that can combine with the body's building blocks (proteins), lipids, and genetic coding material (DNA). The cumulative effects of glucose or glycosylation reactions with proteins and genetic material have been increasingly implicated in the secondary problems of diabetes. As has been discussed, the monitoring of glycosylated hemoglobin or HbA_{1c} values has been useful in providing an index of "control" for the person with diabetes. Acetaldehyde has also been found to form relatively stable combinations with these building blocks and genetic material, and further protein modification with acetaldehyde can occur to proteins that have previously reacted with sugar or been glycosylated. The role of these types of combinations in the problems associated with alcohol ingestion is an area of research with important clinical implications. Recent studies show promise. Now there is a test for acetaldehyde reaction products with plasma proteins or hemoglobin, a test that may be useful in assessing alcohol intake in a manner analogous to the use of hemoglobin A_{1c} in diabetes.

The breakdown of glucose and alcohol both change the way a cell uses oxygen. The chemical breakdown pathways of each are determined, in part, by the intracellular concentrations and the presence of other drugs or chemicals. Little information is available concerning the direct interaction of alcohol or its breakdown products on the breakdown of glucose or its metabolism.

Damage to Muscles and Nerves

Both hyperglycemia and alcohol can cause nerve damage (neuropathy) and muscle damage (myopathy) by mechanisms that are only partially understood. Metabolic and/or toxic neuropathies tend to potentiate each other. Therefore, other potential causes of nerve damage, including alcohol-induced vitamin B_{12} deficiency and lead poisoning, need to be eliminated in an individual with diabetes before all symptoms are ascribed to hyperglycemia.

Sexual Dysfunctions

Both diabetes and alcohol can lead to sexual dysfunction. Both are associated with impotence. In addition, both hyperglycemia and alcohol have a direct toxic effect on the reproductive glands, especially the testes. Levels of male hormone (testosterone) but not female hormone (estradiol) are suppressed in acute and chronic alcohol abuse. Nonetheless, reproductive changes are seen in alcoholic women as well, including menstrual disturbances, loss of secondary sex characteristics, and infertility. Therefore, alcohol would appear to worsen the sexual dysfunction associated with the blood vessel, and nerve changes seen in diabetes.

Heart Problems

Risk of heart attacks and strokes increases with diabetes and with alcohol abuse. The relative and somewhat controversial protective effect of alcohol at low doses is lost at higher doses. In addition, alcohol intake is associated with high blood pressure and an increase in blood fats (cholesterol and triglycerides). If you are a hypertensive, hyperlipidemic and have diabetes (high sugar, high fat, and high blood pressure), you must stop drinking alcohol if these risks are to be minimized.

Diseases of the Bloodstream

Hyperglycemia also predisposes the blood to clotting. Thus, it would appear that the coexistence of high glucose and alcohol would predispose a person to strokes as well as generalized vascular disease. Alcohol is also directly toxic to brain function and the heart.

Liver Problems

The liver is the primary site of alcohol breakdown. Alcohol abuse can cause changes to the liver in the form of fatty liver, alcoholic hepatitis, or cirrhosis; these changes can occur even in the absence of poor eating habits. These liver changes make the person with diabetes increasingly vulnerable to hypoglycemia and acidosis as noted above. Diabetes out of control can result in a fatty liver even without the addition of too much alcohol.

Eye Problems

There is an increased prevalence of cataracts in alcoholic and diabetic individuals. Combination of small molecules with proteins and changes in the state of the lens tissue have been implicated in the cataracts of aging, diabetes, and alcohol intake.

Susceptibility to Infectious Diseases

Chronic alcohol abuse and diabetes are associated with enhanced susceptibility to several infectious diseases. This association suggests that the body's ability to recognize or fight viruses and bacteria is severely compromised by both alcohol and hyperglycemia. In individuals who are hyperglycemic or who have abused alcohol, the white blood cells that fight infection show several defects.

Skin and Bone Changes

Skin and bone changes occur in both diabetes and alcoholism. Studies of alcoholics and diabetics have indicated a reduction in bone mass (or osteoporosis) in various parts of the body. While osteoporosis is generally considered a problem of women, drinking alcohol has also been implicated as a risk factor for osteoporosis in men.

Pregnancy Complications

The risk to the unborn child is increased by both alcohol and hyperglycemia. The risk is not only confined to increased rates of miscarriage and malformations in the first trimester. Miscarriage, stillbirths, and premature births are increased in both diseases. Therefore, the avoidance of even minimal elevations of glucose and total avoidance of alcohol are advocated during pregnancy.

Gastrointestinal Disorders

Gastroparesis, or immobility of the stomach, is an infrequent but devastating consequence of diabetes. Degenerative changes in the vagus nerve that controls the stomach have been described in both diabetic and alcoholic subjects. Alcohol intake is associated with impaired mobility, inflammation of the lining of the gut, and other gastrointestinal disorders.

Work-Related Problems

Finally, securing and maintaining employment are difficult enough for the person with diabetes. The drinking diabetic often has increased work-related problems. Disruptions in job and family caused by drinking add to the stress of having diabetes, blur the judgment, and ultimately may overwhelm the coping capabilities of even the strongest individual.

WHAT IF YOU DECIDE TO DRINK ANYWAY?

Despite the above, you may decide to experiment with alcoholic beverages or to continue drinking. The following outlines an approach to drinking for type 1 or insulin-using type 2 persons who may be drinking alcoholic beverages for the first time (more than about 30 grams of alcohol, or the equivalent of two glasses of wine) or for sporadic "social" drinking.

1. Chart food, drinks, and glucose.
2. Check your blood glucose before and one hour after starting drinking.
3. Check your blood glucose before going to bed.
4. If taking insulin, cut your nighttime NPH or intermediate insulin by one-half.
5. Check your blood glucose at 3:00 A.M. and correct hypoglycemia if necessary with food.
6. Check your blood glucose at your normal wake-up time and "touch up" with food or insulin based on the results.

You should realize that alcohol is a dangerous drug, and therefore planning for drinking and strict surveillance of blood glucose levels are required if problems are to be avoided. Checking blood sugar levels before and after the start of drinking (and eating) will allow you to learn the effect of a particular beverage on blood glucose levels. The subsequent blood sugar checks at bedtime, 3:00 A.M., and in the morning are designed to monitor the longer-term hypoglycemic effects of alcohol in order to avoid harm.

Although alcohol is not usually on the meal plan for a person with diabetes, diabetic persons can occasionally have a drink if they drink in moderation and adjust their diabetes program appropriately. If you are going to try alcohol, it is helpful if you are using either an intermediate acting insulin (NPH or Lente) plus Regular, Lispro, or a pump. With any of these insulin regimens, the overnight insulin dose can be safely cut in half. If Ultralente is being used to cover basal insulin needs, the cost can be cut in half for overnight coverage, but insulin levels do not drop as rapidly in response to the dose decrease, and hence the vulnerability to hypoglycemia is greater. Furthermore, there is a greater possibility with Ultralente that the insulin dose may have been taken before "unanticipated drinking" occurs.

Each person is sensitive to somewhat different doses of alcohol in terms of the potential hypoglycemic effect of the drug. In addition, "tolerance" to alcohol occurs, so that the dose required for a hypoglycemic effect varies with exposure. Therefore, it is best to err "on the safe side" regarding insulin requirements for those who wish to drink.

What about the person with type 2 diabetes who wishes to drink? In this case, the caloric content of alcohol (7 calories per gram or about as much as pure fat) becomes an important factor, since a weight-loss program is easily sabotaged with alcohol. Furthermore, if oral agents such as sulfonylureas are being used for diabetes management, an inhibition of alcohol breakdown by these agents may result in elevated levels of acetaldehyde in the bloodstream following alcohol ingestion. This can lead to increased flushing, especially in the face, but sometimes over the whole body after as little as a single drink. Elevated levels of acetaldehyde result in symptoms including malaise, flushing, feeling feverish, and at times itching, nausea, and vomiting—similar to the interaction of alcohol and the drug Antabuse, which is prescribed to help some alcoholics avoid drinking.

The dangers of using an oral hypoglycemic agent in an alcoholic person generally outweighs the potential benefits, and a drinking problem should first be corrected before oral hypoglycemic agents are used. Insulin use as outlined above can be helpful as a temporary measure to lower blood glucose levels while drinking continues. In view of the risks of hypoglycemia cited above, the target levels of blood glucose for a diabetic person with a drinking problem need to be at a somewhat higher level (for example, 100–200 mg/dl) than for the nondrinking person.

7

Your Exercise Program

Charlotte was diagnosed as having diabetes at age ten. Now in her late twenties, she has injected her insulin once a day. She did not have her eyes checked for several years and was alarmed to wake up one morning with spots in her right eye. A visit to an eye doctor revealed a ruptured blood vessel in the back of the retina, which left a blood deposit between the lens and retina in the area called the vitreous humor.

To save her sight, Charlotte underwent a series of laser treatments (photocoagulation). After each treatment, she was advised to rest at home for about two weeks and remain still. She was not allowed to lift anything or bend over, since these actions would put pressure on her eyes. With time on her hands, Charlotte began to measure her urine glucose levels throughout the day. They were usually about 0.75 percent in the morning but rose to 2 percent later, with some ketone spilling into her urine. When her hemoglobin A_{1c} measured 12 percent, Charlotte's doctor recommended strict diabetes control and the use of a self-monitoring meter to keep track of her blood glucose levels. Because of her eye problem, Charlotte was afraid to exercise. Four months after her last laser treatment, she was allowed to start some simple *conditioning and stretching exercises. She used a stationary bicycle at home and later moved into more strenuous exercises, still careful not to do heavy weightlifting. Two years later her eye condition had stabilized and her hemoglobin A_{1c} was in the normal range for over a year. She is now in better physical condition than ever and continues a health maintenance program of insulin, proper food, and exercise.*

Charlotte's case demonstrates the importance of exercise to help lower blood glucose levels. Exercise appears to help transport glucose out of your bloodstream and into the cells where it can be used. The more you exercise, the more glucose you use. Also, the harder you exercise, the faster the glucose is transported to your cells.

Exercise also builds muscle tone. In addition to becoming firmer and stronger, your muscles will acquire more glycogen, the substance in which glucose is stored. This protects you against hypoglycemic attacks. When your blood glucose drops too low, your body mobilizes glycogen to bring glucose into your bloodstream. The better conditioning you maintain, the more protection you have against hypoglycemia. The more glycogen stored in your liver and muscles, the better prepared you are to combat a hypoglycemic episode without plummeting to a dangerous low.

Basically, there are three types of exercises: those that condition, those that build strength, and those that increase flexibility (see Table 7.1). Conditioning (or endurance) exercises include bicycling, swimming, and jogging—all of which bring your heart rate above 120 beats per minute. You should maintain your pulse at this rate or higher for periods of at least twenty minutes to get a good conditioning effect. This will increase the ability of your heart to work without strain and improve your overall cardiovascular performance. The muscles do not necessarily get big-

TABLE 7.1 Types of Exercise

Conditioning	Flexibility	Strength
Walking	Stretching	Body Building
Jogging	Yoga	Weightlifting
Running	Calisthenics	Nautilus Training
Cycling		
Tennis		
Swimming		
Rope Jumping		
Skiing		
Ice Skating		
Roller Skating		
Rowing		
Climbing		

ger in conditioning exercises, but they do get stronger and have less fat.

Strength-building or resistance exercises increase muscle bulk as well as tone and strength. The most common type is weightlifting. As in Charlotte's case, persons with retinal disease should avoid strength-training exercises until the retina heals.

The more you exercise and increase your flexibility and endurance, the better you will feel. To be truly effective, you should exercise at least three times a week, preferably on alternate days. As your condition improves, it will require more and harder exercise to raise your pulse rate above 120 and keep it there for twenty minutes. Also, if you are in good condition, your pulse beat will return more quickly to its normal resting rate. Your resting pulse rate will also be somewhat slower if you are in good condition.

To evaluate your present physical status, you can undergo endurance strength and flexibility tests at your local Y or some similar program. An inexpensive and accessible way to assess your physical condition is to run up and down a flight of twelve stairs

TABLE 7.2 Evaluating Your Physical Condition

Your physical condition can be judged by how long it takes your pulse to return to normal after strenuous activity, such as running up and down stairs.

Good	1 minute
Fair	3 minutes
Poor	4–5 minutes
Need Help	over 5 minutes

at least five times. Measure your pulse rate before you start and then again when you finish. Obviously, the better your condition, the faster you will complete this exercise. You should also note how long it takes your pulse rate to return to the level it was before you ran up and down the stairs. If your pulse rate is back to normal in one minute, you are in good condition; in three minutes, fair; four to five minutes, poor; and longer than five minutes, you need help (see Table 7.2).

In addition to toning your muscles and firming your body, proper exercise benefits you in other ways that are especially important. Exercise increases the blood flow to all your body's organs and helps your muscles use glucose independently of insulin. The increased blood flow expands your blood vessels, which is especially important for persons with diabetes since they are prone to narrowed vessels. Exercise aids in metabolizing fats in your bloodstream, consequently lowering your cholesterol and triglyceride levels.

An exercise program should be calculated to fit your general situation and should be increased at a slow but steady rate. Sports trainers and exercise experts do this automatically with athletic teams, and it takes about three months to get them in optimum condition. You should expect no less for yourself.

When you do a relatively fixed amount of daily exercise and increase it gradually, you can begin to calibrate what exercise does to your blood glucose levels. You should measure your blood glucose before you exercise, immediately after, and an hour later. As you increase the amount of exercise, you will find that blood glucose levels are lowered by increasing amounts, and you will want to know what this amount is. When you are not in good condition, for example, thirty minutes of exercise may only lower your blood glucose 10 mg/dl. In fact, if you are in poor physical condition, your sugars may rise from the "stress" of exercise. Also if your glucose levels are too high when you start exercise, they may rise further. As your physical condition peaks, this same amount of exercise may lower your blood glucose by as much as 60 mg/dl. Moreover, the blood glucose may continue to go down up to five hours after you have finished exercising. In other words, when you are in good physical condition, you can almost use exercise as you do Regular insulin, on top of your long-acting insulin, to lower your blood glucose immediately. If you are in excellent condition, you can even calibrate your exercise as you do insulin to substitute exercise for insulin.

There is an easier way to control your blood glucose during exercise. Since you can't always determine the exact time and amount of exercise you will be doing, you can use those fast-acting sugars you calibrated earlier with your exercise and not jeopardize your blood glucose. When you know what a given amount of exercise does to your blood glucose level, you will be able to calculate how much fruit juice or fresh fruit you need to maintain your blood glucose within the normal range. For example, if your starting blood glucose is normal and you take a small amount of juice or fast-acting sugar immediately before exercising, and the same amount every ten minutes while exercising, you will have a normal blood glucose upon completing the exercise period.

You must beware, however, not to lower your blood glucose further during the time following exercise. During a tennis game, for example, you can have a jar of diluted orange juice by the net and drink some each time you finish a game to keep yourself at normal levels. This is known as "anticipating exercise with calories" to maintain your blood glucose at optimum levels during the exercise period.

If you are not trained or fit, it is better to avoid strenuous exercise when your glucose is above 300 mg/dl. Your glucose should not be going anywhere near this high, but if you exercise at this level your performance will be poor. In addition, exercise at this high level of blood glucose tends to lead to the accumulation of extra lactic acid in the blood. Therefore, it is important to maintain good control even with exercise!

The best way to keep in shape is to have an established exercise program such as stationary cycling or jogging. This permits your to stay in condition from day to day in a relatively efficient way with perhaps thirty minutes to an hour of exercise three or more days a week. It also gives you a predictable program that you can incorporate into your diabetic regimen (Table 7.3). Because of its predictability, you can often decrease your insulin or medication dosage just prior to your exercise period. So you have two insulin or medication regimens: one for exercise days and

TABLE 7.3 The Ideal Program

Frequency:	At least three times per week
Warm-up:	3–5 minutes
Conditioning:	20–30 minutes
Flexibility exercise or "fun" games such as volleyball:	10–15 minutes
Strength training:	According to physician's recommendations
Slow, steady progress:	Most training programs take about 3–6 months to reach maximum fitness

one for other days. Sports and other athletic activities are less predictable than established exercises, and you may have to anticipate this type of exercise with calories to maintain your blood glucose.

By using your glucose meter and calibrating foods, you will soon achieve another degree of freedom in controlling your diabetes through exercise. You need no longer be afraid of strenuous activities or exercise. In fact, you will know they are good for you. You will feel better because you are taking better care of your body, and your body will appreciate it. Your muscles will begin to firm up and your posture will improve. A bonus benefit is an increased energy level, with less fatigue and improved bodily functions. Along with your physical health, exercise aids your mental health and provides a sense of general well-being.

Strength training is also becoming increasingly popular. Strength training has been shown to have a glucose-lowering effect and to decrease insulin requirements over time just as cardiovascular conditioning does. The major difference between cardiovascular conditioning and strength training is that strength training may not lead to an acute drop in blood glucose levels during the workout. Cardiovascular conditioning routines drop blood glucose during the workout depending on the level of conditioning. Even unfit persons with diabetes who start a cardiovascular conditioning program three times per week will begin to notice an acute lowering of blood glucose after about the sixth workout. Therefore, if you want to lower your blood glucose with exercise, use a cardiovascular conditioning workout. If you are already in the normal range and don't want to consume extra sugar in order to work out, use a strength training routine.

Before you start a strength training program, it is a good idea to discuss it with your doctor. Strength exercises are associated with an increase in blood pressure, which may put additional stresses on the heart and small vessels of the eyes during the workout. Therefore it is important to make sure that these systems are "go" before starting on this type of exercise routine.

Persons with diabetes who take up strength training are often curious about the use of anabolic steroids. These drugs can make for bulky muscles, but they are a health disaster for anyone, especially for someone with diabetes. Steroids not only cause liver damage, acne, and alter sexual functions and emotions, they also raise blood sugar. Therefore, the person with diabetes should definitely avoid anabolic steroids.

There is one drug available to the diabetic individual (and no one else) which does help build muscle tissue. That drug is insulin. When used correctly to control blood sugar, insulin also helps build muscles.

As discussed in the next chapter, even pregnant women can use exercise to help manage their diabetes. It is not necessary to become a "jock" or "fitness freak" to appreciate the benefits of exercise. Twenty minutes invested as little as three times per week can make a huge difference.

As always, remember the key to what you are doing is to measure what effect a given variable has on you and your blood glucose. When in doubt, check your blood glucose because that will give you the number you need to respond appropriately to any problem. Remember, get a program you enjoy and look forward to. This is the best way to "stick with it" and get the most benefit over time.

8

Pregnancy and Diabetes

emember Ann? She was the
patient we discussed in Chap-
ter 3. She decided to decrease her insulin as she decreased her
food. Ann has been working hard to keep her glycosylated hemoglobin in the normal range. Not only does she feel better when
she keeps herself in control, but she and her husband plan to have
a baby soon, and she wants to be in the best health possible.

The evidence is clear that high blood glucose levels at the time
of conception may cause birth defects in the baby. No one knows
the exact mechanism whereby hyperglycemia may cause birth
defects; however, we can understand that the rapidly dividing
cells forming organs would not like to divide in a sticky sugar
environment. The safest advice at the moment is for a diabetic
woman to plan pregnancy and become pregnant when her glycosylated hemoglobin is in the normal range.

WILL YOUR BABY BE BORN WITH DIABETES?

Although diabetes may not be the worst problem in the world to
have, you certainly would be grateful if your child did not have it.
The type of diabetes which your baby might inherit from you

will be your type of diabetes. If you got your diabetes at age eight, then your child's diabetes would be type 1 diabetes. And, it is exceedingly rare for a baby to be born with diabetes! The chances that your child will get diabetes at all depends not only on your genes but also on whether your husband is carrying the gene for diabetes. It would be a good idea to ask your husband and his family about forgotten grandmothers, aunts, uncles, or cousins who may have had diabetes. Diabetes affects 5 percent of the population in the United States. Therefore, if you look hard enough, you may find that you and your husband share a genetic predisposition to diabetes.

If only you carry the gene, and if you have type 1 diabetes, no more than one in four of your children will inherit the gene. This does not mean that 25 percent of your children will get diabetes, however, for manifestation of the disease requires not only a genetic predisposition to diabetes but also an environmental factor such as a viral infection. Furthermore, the inheritance of diabetes requires more than one gene for most kinds of diabetes. Therefore, the true chances that your child will develop diabetes are less than 6 percent, if you have type 1 diabetes.

If you have type 2 diabetes, the probability that your child will inherit your diabetic gene goes up, but here, again, environment plays a big role and, of course, this type of diabetes presents in adulthood. If that child stays lean and fit, even with the genetic vulnerability, it may be possible to avoid the problem. If you have type 1 diabetes and your husband has type 2 diabetes in his family, your child could inherit one or both of these traits.

Whether or not you might pass the gene to your child should not influence your decision to have children. For the truth is that no one really knows what the chances are that your particular children will develop diabetes. Thus, it is unlikely that you will see diabetes in your child. There are some rare exceptions where the inheritance is more prevalent and is generally about 50 percent. If you think you might have one of these rare forms of diabetes such as Maturity Onset Diabetes of Youth (MODY), Atypical Diabetes Mellitus (ADM) of the young, or maternal linked mitochondrial DNA diabetes in one of its forms, discuss the issue of inheritance with your physician.

PLANNING A PREGNANCY

If your glycosylated hemoglobin is normal, then the outlook for pregnancy is good. However, your health should also be checked concerning the status of your eyes, kidneys, and blood pressure. Although it has been shown that a woman with normal blood glucose levels will produce a normal baby, retinopathy, nephropathy (kidney disease), and hypertension could complicate a pregnancy as well as present risk factors for the mother and the baby. In fact, a classification of pregnancies based on complications of the mother takes into account the health of the mother before she becomes pregnant. Have your eye doctor reassure you that your retina is healthy and have your kidneys and blood pressure checked as well.

This does not mean that you should not become pregnant if you have had laser therapy for your retinas. It does mean that before attempting a pregnancy, there should be no new vessel growth which tends to worsen during pregnancy. Therefore, the time to fix the problem with laser therapy is before pregnancy. Your kidneys are tested by a twenty-four-hour collection of urine paired with a blood test. If there are kidney and/or blood pressure problems, it is best to have these taken care of and controlled for about a year before becoming pregnant. Pregnancy is considered safe for both mother and child if you have at least half your kidney function intact. Hypertension is the greatest risk factor for your pregnancy. If you begin the pregnancy with an elevated blood pressure, then you add the serious problems of hypertension to your pregnancy. The bottom line is that pregnancy should be planned and you should be as healthy as possible to assure a normal healthy baby and mother.

WHAT IS GESTATIONAL DIABETES?

Elaine is a healthy thirty-two-year-old woman who decided to have children after she completed law school and settled in practice. She was never sick a day in her life, but always fought to lose the twenty extra pounds she carried around. During her first pregnancy, she gained twice the weight that her obstetrician advised, but felt well the entire nine months. One week before her due date, she noticed that the baby had stopped kicking. One day later she delivered a 10-pound stillbirth. What happened? Why did Elaine lose her baby?

Several points in Elaine's history made her doctor suspect that Elaine had gestational diabetes—that is, diabetes that is first recognized during pregnancy. First, Elaine's grandmother and aunt have type 2 diabetes mellitus. Second, Elaine herself weighed over nine pounds at birth. Both these points mean that Elaine had a good chance of getting diabetes during her pregnancy.

However, Elaine never experienced the classic signs of diabetes, and her blood sugar levels after the delivery were normal. The definition of gestational diabetes, then, necessitates that the diabetes begins during the pregnancy and goes away after the pregnancy. Elaine's blood glucose levels were not high enough to cause her symptoms but were high enough to kill her unborn child.

How Does High Blood Glucose Kill an Unborn Child?

Maternal sugar crosses the placenta into the baby's bloodstream. The mother's insulin does not cross into the baby. The baby starts to make insulin from the end of the first trimester of the pregnancy onward. When the level of sugar coming from the mother stimulates overproduction of insulin by the baby, the baby becomes fat, lethargic, and metabolically unstable. This metabolic instability may cause death. This problem is completely solved when the mother's blood glucose levels are normal.

What Is Considered Normal Blood Glucose for a Pregnant Woman?

Pregnancy normally confers with it lower blood glucose levels than usual. Therefore, the goal of therapy is to mimic the blood glucose ranges of a normal pregnancy. The normal glucose levels for pregnancy are as follows:

> Fasting = BS 55–65 mg/dl, the maximum value
> 1 hour after a meal < 120 mg/dl and the average
> blood glucose = 80–90 mg/dl

Whether a woman has had diabetes for many years before the pregnancy (pregestational) or gets diabetes during her pregnancy (gestational), her blood glucose levels must be normal to assure a normal outcome. If her blood glucose levels are elevated, then her pregnancy becomes "high-risk" for both her and her unborn child. A pregnancy can therefore be classified by three criteria:

1. Whether the diabetes has its onset before or during pregnancy (pregestational versus gestational diabetes).
2. Whether the mother's blood glucose levels are normal for the entire pregnancy (normal glucose levels versus elevated glucose levels).
3. Whether the woman starts her pregnancy with hypertension.

Screening for Gestational Diabetes

The prevalence of gestational diabetes is as much as 12 percent of all pregnancies in high risk groups such as those of Hispanic origin in the United States. Because undiagnosed gestational diabetes can kill unborn infants, it is absolutely necessary for all pregnant women to have a glucose challenge test in the middle of their pregnancy to test for diabetes. The test requires the woman to drink a perfectly measured sugar drink (50 grams of glucose) and then, one hour later, have a blood test for her glucose level. A urine test for sugar is not sensitive enough to make the diagnosis of gestational diabetes. Only a blood test performed in this fashion can reassure a woman that she does not have diabetes. *All* pregnant women should have this test at twenty-six to twenty-eight weeks of gestation. Those women who have a history of previous big babies, a stillbirth, or a family history of diabetes should have the test even earlier.

If there is suspicion of diabetes (that is, if the one-hour glucose level is > 140 mg/dl), then a three-hour glucose tolerance test is necessary. For the three hour test, blood is drawn after an overnight fast and on an empty stomach, followed by a drink of 100 grams of glucose. The criteria for the diagnosis of gestational diabetes continue to be debated by the experts. The diagnosis of gestational diabetes by the most commonly used criteria is made if the fasting is over 105 mg/dl and/or two of the post-drink blood glucose values are higher than the cutoff points of 195 at one hour, 165 at two hours, and 145 mg/dl at three hours. Others would like to lower the criteria: Dr. Coustan would have a fasting 95, one hour 180, two hours 155, and five hours 140 mg/dl; while Dr. Sacks would have 96, 172, 152, and 131 mg/dl for the respective time points. Regardless of your test outcome, if you suspect your sugars are going too high, you can always check them before and after meals to make sure they are at a healthy level for you and your baby.

If the fasting level is greater than 105, then insulin is immediately necessary to give the patient room to eat and still stay in the normal range. Some consider the level of 105 too high and if the fasting does not come down on diet therapy to a level below 90 mg/dl, we tend to start insulin.

If the fasting is normal but the postdrink results are high, diet therapy alone may succeed in maintaining the mother's blood glucose levels in the normal range. The patient should verify whether her diet is helping her maintain normal glucose levels. She can do this by checking her blood glucose fasting and one hour after a meal. If her blood test reveals that she is high despite compliance to her diet prescription, insulin must be started.

THE DIET PRESCRIPTION

For a normal weight gain in pregnancy, the caloric intake must be increased from 25 calories per kilogram of body weight a day (for a woman of ideal body weight) to 30 calories/kg/day at eight weeks of gestation. For obese women, the calories per kilogram body weight calculation may be much lower such that women who are very obese might require as few as 12 calories/kg/day even when pregnant. To find out the best caloric calculation,

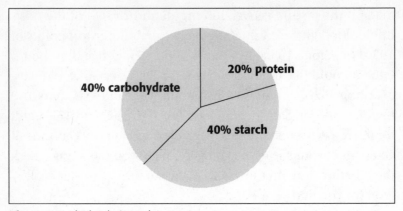

Figure 8.1 Ideal Caloric Intake

consult your health care team experienced in the care of pregnant women with diabetes.

The caloric intake is best divided into 40 percent carbohydrate, 20 percent protein, and 40 percent fat (see Figure 8.1). Breakfast must be small in order for the after-breakfast blood glucose to be normal. In addition, frequent small meals have a better chance of maintaining the blood glucose at normal levels than large meals.

Thus, the calories should be divided so that 12 percent are at breakfast, 30 percent at lunch and dinner, and the rest divided into snacks at midmorning, mid-afternoon, and late evening (Figure 8.2).

If a woman starts her pregnancy overweight, then she needs fewer calories than if she started at a normal weight. For the woman who is greater than 120 percent of her ideal body weight, the diet calorie prescription during pregnancy should be 24 calories/kg/day, divided as in Table 8.2 into three meals and three to four snacks. As noted above, women who are even heavier may require even fewer calories.

The diet for a gestational diabetic woman is the key to normal blood glucose levels and thus a normal baby. The woman

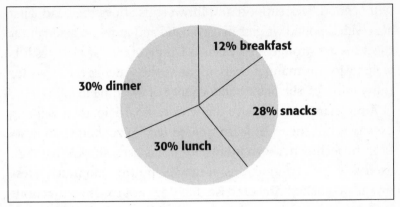

Figure 8.2 Ideal Caloric Breakdown

with gestational diabetes needs to measure her blood glucose level at least four times a day: before breakfast and one hour after each meal. If her fasting level is above 90 mg/dl, then she needs to take NPH before bed to help her lower her wake-up blood glucose the next morning. If her blood glucose levels are above 140 mg/dl one hour after the meal, then she can first try decreasing the carbohydrate content of the meal plan. Eliminating the bread or potato usually does the trick. If this does not work, then the woman must also take a short-acting insulin before each meal.

One other option besides insulin therapy is available for the gestational diabetic woman when she notes that her blood glucose levels are high despite changes in her diet. This option is an exercise program. The only way to burn excess sugar is to exert energy. The safest exercise program for a gestational diabetic woman may be swimming. Swimming is gentle on the abdominal muscles and uses energy by forcing the arms to do most of the work. Weight-bearing exercises and bicycling are sometimes too strenuous for the mother, irritating the womb and starting contractions, thus putting stress on the baby. Arm exercises do not cause any of these problems. Another suggestion is to sit in a chair with a good back support and lift weights above the head. First start with 2-pound weights in each hand and move up gradually as the arms get stronger. If a woman with gestational diabetes lifts weights in this manner every night as she watches the news for thirty minutes, she has a better chance of avoiding insulin.

A pregnant woman with diabetes can participate in walking exercises, but she must learn how to recognize uterine contractions by feeling her own uterus, for it has been shown that if an exercise causes contractions, it may be putting too much stress on the pregnancy. Any exercise that does not cause contractions is therefore safe. Thus, self-uterine monitoring has also become a part of pregnancy management.

Elaine—the woman who had gestational diabetes—became pregnant again. At twenty-six weeks of gestation she had a glucose challenge test; the result was 180 mg/dl. On the next day she underwent the three-hour test. Her fasting blood glucose was 85, but all other glucose levels were higher than the cutoff. Elaine was able to keep all her after-meal blood glucose levels normal with the diet prescription, and she delivered a healthy 7½-pound baby.

The Need for Insulin in Gestational Diabetes

If the blood glucose levels of a pregnant woman cannot be maintained in the normal range, then insulin is necessary. The insulin prescription not only should be calculated according to her present pregnant weight but also should take into account her weeks of gestation (see Table 8.1).

NPH is a better choice for pregnancy than Ultralente because Ultralente is hard to adjust upward quickly as the baby grows. The total insulin requirement is then divided in the same fashion as discussed in Chapter 3. Whether the woman is a gestational or pregestational diabetic patient, the above calculations apply. In-

TABLE 8.1 Normal Range of Glucose During Pregnancy

Week of Gestation	Insulin Requirement (NPH Family)
1st day of missed period to week 18	0.7 units/kg/24 hours
Weeks 18–28	0.8
Weeks 28–36	0.9
Weeks 36–40	1.0

sulin is the best drug for diabetes during pregnancy. Unlike the medicine in pills, insulin generally does not cross the placenta and hence cannot harm the baby. Glucose, on the other hand, does cross the placenta and can harm the baby as can many of the drugs that are used for treating diabetes.

AS THE BIG MOMENT APPROACHES . . .

As long as the mother's blood glucose levels are normal, the baby should be normal. To make sure that all goes well, you and your baby will begin to undergo tests when you reach the last third of your pregnancy. Your obstetrician will ask you to keep track of the number of baby kicks you feel in one hour, every day at the same time. The more your baby kicks, the healthier your baby seems to be. If the number of baby kicks decreases, you should notify your doctor.

Because you have kept your blood glucose levels normal, your baby should not be too fat. Previously, all diabetic women were often advised to have a cesarean section to deliver their over-sized infants. Now you should be able to deliver the normal way, unless your obstetrician recommends a cesarean section for other reasons.

During labor, your insulin needs will drop. This drop happens in part because labor is a form of exercise. Once labor starts, do not take your next injection of insulin. Call your doctor immediately and ask what to do and when you should come to the hospital. The exercise of your labor may lower your blood glucose level. You probably will need glucose solutions by vein to give you energy for childbirth.

AFTER CHILDBIRTH

Once you have given birth, you get a breather; after the baby is born your insulin requirement generally will remain very low for twenty-four to seventy-two hours. If you had gestational diabetes, the need for insulin will have gone away. But be forewarned—there is a 95 percent chance of the gestational diabetes recurring in every subsequent pregnancy.

Do you want to breast-feed? Of course, you can breast-feed. You will need to keep your diet rich in calcium, but you will find that your overnight need for insulin will decrease depending on how much the baby drinks overnight. Don't worry about insulin appearing in the breast milk—it will not be absorbed by the baby's bloodstream. If insulin could be absorbed when ingested with milk, then you, too, could drink your insulin in milk. Your blood glucose level does affect the milk sugar content, however. If you are concerned about your baby drinking too much sweet milk, then it is best to keep your blood sugar normal for as long as you breast-feed.

Although the effort for you as a pregnant diabetic person was greater than any nondiabetic person can imagine, the glorious birth of a healthy baby is well worth the investment.

9

Travel

Bon voyage! Have a good trip! These hopeful words of departure can come true for the diabetic traveler who prepares wisely for the adventure. There are three important points to remember and plan for before leaving on a trip.

1. Take enough supplies with you so that you do not need to search for a pharmacy in a strange place. The rule of thumb is to take *twice* as much insulin and twice as many syringes, wipes, and test strips as you would normally need and carry them in two different places (see Table 9.1).

2. Carry a letter explaining the reason for your supplies, signed by a nurse or physician. If you are going abroad, there is a possibility that you may be questioned about your medications and syringes. Although there is no law that a diabetic person must justify his or her supplies at a border control station, why risk a possible, though unlikely, encounter with a suspicious inspector?

3. Take time changes into account. If John is planning to cross time zones, then he must consider two changes. The first is the loss or addition of hours in the day. An extreme example would be a nonstop trip from California to London, which would result in the loss of eight hours on the travel day. Thus, John would merely skip his before-bed NPH injection, for it is an eight-hour insulin. On the airplane, he would probably be fed twice; thus he would need to take two injections of Regular to cover the two meals. Coming back, he would add eight hours to his day, and therefore he should repeat his bedtime dose eight hours after his usual NPH injection at the origin of the day's travel, to come back into California time. Thus, for each desti-

Table 9.1 Sample Travel Supplies for Two Weeks

John is going to Cape Cod for two weeks. He uses one syringe a day for his three injections, tests his blood glucose five times a day, and uses 30 units of NPH and 18 units of Regular a day. Therefore, he should bring the following with him:

Syringes	1 syringe × 14 days × 2 (in case) = 28 syringes
NPH	30 units/day × 14 days × 2 (in case) = 840 units (Each bottle of NPH contains 1,000 units, so one bottle would be enough. But what if that bottle breaks? Better take two bottles.)
Regular	18 units/day × 14 days × 2 (in case) = 504 units (One bottle of Regular contains 1,000 units. To be sure, and to give John extra insulin to splurge on large vacation meals, he'd better take two bottles.)
Wipes	3 injections/day + 5 blood glucose tests/day × 14 days × 2 (in case) = 224 wipes. (Each box has 200 wipes. Better take two boxes.)
Test strips	5 tests/day × 14 days × 2 (in case) = 140 strips (If each bottle contains 25 strips, then John needs 6 bottles.)

nation, the time there compared with the time at home must be known in order to derive the formula for travel.

The second change that needs to be understood is the problem known as jet lag. The body has its own internal "clock," set according to the rhythm of a rest-activity cycle and a body-temperature cycle. These cycles affect your energy levels at various times of the day and your needs for insulin. When you are at home, your internal clock is synchronized with local time. Your body can tolerate westbound travel because a fall back in time does not affect its rhythm as much as a skip ahead in time. If your destination is more than two hours behind or one hour ahead, your energy level is high or low at the "wrong" time.

The reason you, as a person with diabetes, should understand these daily rhythms is that your overnight need for insulin is significantly different from your usual daytime needs. Thus, at 3:00 A.M. in California, John would need very little insulin, but from 3:00 A.M. to 10:00 A.M. he would need a lot of insulin to keep his blood glucose normal. In London, this high insulin need stays on "California time" for about a week and therefore is pushed up to the period 11:00 A.M. to 7:00 P.M. John could increase his lunchtime and dinner Regular to cover this increased need. But he should be cautioned that if he stays more than five days to a week in London, his inner clock will reset to London time, and so 3:00 A.M. becomes 3:00 A.M. again as far as his body is concerned. He will then need to readjust when he returns home because his body will stay on London time for about the same five to seven days.

One last word of caution about traveling: carry enough pocket food to treat a low blood sugar. Because your internal clock is changing slowly to adjust to the abrupt time change, your insulin needs may not be predictable. Insulin may act stronger than it usually does, so taking pocket food along is a must. In a foreign place, trying to speak another language and make a purchase with foreign money is a tough enough task, let alone during an insulin reaction.

The exercise level of a traveler is also unpredictable. The travel itself may be no exercise (as in the case of car, train, or plane) or all exercise (as in the case of bicycle riding or a strenuous hike with luggage). In addition, on some days all sightseeing may be done on a bus, on other days all on foot. Pocket food comes in handy for the days when exercise turns out to be more than anticipated by a morning dose of insulin. Of course, it would be wise to carry a syringe with Regular in it or an insulin pen in order to take extra insulin on days with little exercise—or in case the tour bus stops in front of the best pastry shop in all of Europe.

10

Problem Situations

ILLNESS

Sometimes diabetes is expensive to manage because even a common cold may require medical attention. Your metabolic needs increase during illness, and often more insulin is required. As you begin to feel poorly, you slow down your activities and burn less glucose. To make matters worse, you lose your appetite and take in fewer calories. In turn, you may be afraid to take your usual insulin dose during illness.

With a split dose or basal bolus insulin plan, or an insulin pump, you are equipped to deal with these situations. Even if you are too ill to eat, you should take your long-acting insulin (or basal rate insulin) to cover your basic metabolic needs. You can continue to monitor your blood glucose levels during the day and use your calibrated short acting insulin to lower rising glucose levels. If you do feel like eating, then you inject short acting insulin before the meal, in addition to your other doses. Remember that glucagon may be used to raise your blood glucose levels, if it becomes necessary. You should contact your physician immediately if you are too ill to monitor your own blood glucose levels or if you are vomiting and cannot eat.

If it appears that you have more than a cold and possibly a bacterial infection, you should also contact your doctor. When it comes to treating a common cold, your doctor's recommendations may do no better or worse than Grandmother's home remedies; but with bacterial infections and the like, the difference can be significant, so do seek medical treatment in such cases.

DENTISTRY

Joan had a very bad toothache. She just made a dental appointment with the dentist's receptionist, who advised her not to eat or drink before her appointment. After she hung up, she realized that complying with this dictum would mean disrupting her insulin schedule. What should Joan do? Should she eat despite the request not to? Of course not, for the advice was meant to make the dental procedure easier and safer. Therefore, Joan should change her insulin dose so that she can skip a meal.

Skipping meals would be easy for Joan if she uses an insulin infusion pump. The pump is programmed to give Joan just enough insulin to keep her normal when she does not eat. If she is taking NPH and Regular in the manner described in Chapter 3, then her bedtime NPH dose is designed to keep her normal for the eight hours of sleep during which she does not eat. Therefore, the bedtime dose of NPH for Joan has been adjusted to fit her needs perfectly. However, if she was not on this system before, a close fit would be calculated as follows: 0.1 × weight in kilograms = NPH dose for fasting. This dose can be repeated every eight hours and adjusted upward or downward depending on the blood glucose levels achieved.

As it turned out, Joan had to go all day without eating, but she succeeded in maintaining her blood glucose at 70–150 mg/dl all day long, and as a bonus she lost two pounds!

SURGERY

Once Joan had learned how to go a whole day without eating, she immediately knew what to do when her dermatologist suggested that she have a mole removed. For this elective surgery, she would take her bedtime NPH the morning of the procedure. Actually, for all elective surgery, this dose of insulin works remarkably well. It may not be enough insulin, however, for the anxiety involved in anticipating surgery may increase the insulin requirement. If the blood glucose levels are 150 mg/dl despite this dose of insulin, one may increase the NPH dose by 2 units or add 2 units of short acting insulin. Frequent blood glucose checks should be made to keep the blood glucose levels normal by adjusting the dose of insulin.

EMERGENCIES

Now let's consider the case of Jill, who had a sudden onset of severe side pain. In the rush to the hospital, she forgot to take her blood-testing material. Upon arrival at the emergency room, Jill was taken to the operating room to stop internal bleeding. In this case of emergency, attention was appropriately placed on correcting the life-threatening problem and not on whether Jill's blood glucose level was normal prior to surgery. Once she was safely in the operating and recovery room, then the attention was refocused on her blood glucose control. Although normal blood glucose is always desirable, it is sometimes necessary to proceed with emergency care despite elevated blood glucose levels.

MISSED MEALS

There will be other times besides dentistry or surgery when you cannot eat at your scheduled mealtime. You may be caught in traffic, at someone's home or school, or in some other set of circumstances that will delay your meal. You should always be prepared with some quick-acting sugar that will tide you over. It is also helpful to have a 40 percent carbohydrate nutrition bar, some cheese, or other protein-containing snack on hand to carry you through even longer situations.

When you do have to vary your mealtime, you might take your long-acting insulin at the usual time with a small protein snack and then, just before you go out or are about to eat, take your short-acting dose. Above all, be prepared to cope with a low blood glucose level. When you do need to miss a meal for any reason, eliminate your short-acting insulin before the skipped meal. You may have to take a bit of quick-acting sugar to compensate, but the only real side effect will be that you end up a little hungry.

EATING OUT

Persons with diabetes need not give up the pleasure of dining out. The major pitfalls are the large food portions served by most restaurants. If you eat out too often, this can lead to excess weight gain. You will probably also need to increase your insulin to accommodate the large quantities. Many people take their premeal Regular insulin after they have looked at the menu and decided what they want to eat. Otherwise, depending on how long you have to wait for your food, you may need a quick-acting sugar to cope with a plummeting blood glucose level. In time you will become quite expert in calculating calories and exchanges from a menu. This ability will see you through many social situations when you are invited to eat out and will enable you to have more freedom in selecting your meal. These situations are where a pump or the shorter acting lispro insulin are helpful. For example, if you have a child with diabetes, you can actually count the carbohydrates your child eats and give lispro afterward and still get reasonable coverage with the insulin dose. With the pump, you can always "touch up" or "graze and bolus" as you decide what you want to eat.

Once you can master carbohydrate counting and insulin matching, eating out should pose no problem. You will have to resist some temptations, however, such as rich desserts, but these are not good for you anyway. If, three hours after your meal, you find that you have overdone it in terms of eating, you can take your calibrated insulin to lower your blood glucose. At worst, your glucose will have been high for a few hours, but you will have avoided a situation in which you are out of phase for days before your glucose calms down.

LOSING WEIGHT

Many diabetic persons want or need to lose weight but get into difficulty because they approach it in a manner that conflicts with a rigid meal and medication plan. The only way to lose weight is to cut calories. For every extra 3,500 calories you eat, you gain another pound of fat. Exercise helps, but it is difficult to lose weight through exercise alone. You simply cannot burn up 3,500 calories in an exercise session unless you are a professional athlete.

Exercise will tone your muscles and put you in better physical condition, but the key to losing weight is fewer calories. For the person with diabetes, fewer calories also means less insulin.

Do not attempt to lose weight too rapidly. During the first week, weight loss is mostly water and not fat. To embark on a sensible weight loss program, reduce your calories by about 10 percent and distribute them evenly throughout the day. You will need to cut your mealtime insulin by approximately the same percentage and distribute your doses in the same manner. You will then begin to burn up fat instead of food and lose about one to three pounds per week. By the end of a month, you will have lost five to ten pounds, an amount recommended for a safe, successful weight loss program. You may feel somewhat hungry at first, but you can sometimes numb the pangs with an exercise session, which will also help change the fat you do have into muscle.

If you modify your eating habits slowly, rather than going on a crash diet, these better eating habits will stay with you, and you will be less apt to regain weight when you have reached your goal.

Some people with type 2 diabetes find that it is impossible for them to eat small meals. They would prefer to avoid food completely rather than trying to have self-control once they start eating. In fact, overeating may be as addictive as a drug or alcohol. These people may need to deal with overeating as an addiction, which includes getting medical and psychological support to overcome the eating disorder. But it is also true that anyone who is overweight has become overweight by overeating. One way to stop the habit of overeating is to stop eating.

Under medical supervision, modified fasting programs have proved to be successful for the diabetic overweight patient. These programs must be undertaken *only with supervision*, because a fast can lead to a dangerous disruption in important blood minerals. In addition, appropriate changes must be made in the diabetes-related medications if a fast is attempted. Usually a patient is allowed to try fasting if he or she is not taking diuretics, does not have heart disease, has normal blood mineral levels, and is on an oral diabetes agent. The oral diabetes agent is stopped the night before the fast, then for two days no food or beverage containing calories is allowed. The person can consume all the water and no-calorie beverages desired. After two days, the patient has a checkup and blood tests to assure that the fast is safe. A two-week rest (resuming normal eating) is usually recommended, then the patient is allowed to try to fast for three days at a time. If the checkup after the three days reveals that the fast is safe, the patient is allowed to fast for three days every two weeks. Usually, 2 to 5 pounds is lost at each fast, so by three months a 15 to 30-pound weight loss is possible! Of course, the only way the fast works is if the patient does not regain weight between the fasts. Thus the fast may need to be a permanent part of management unless general eating patterns are changed.

SMOKING

A diabetic person who smokes is really asking for trouble. Smoking has been linked to vascular disorders, heart disease, and cancer. The combination with diabetes increases the first two risks. For example, 90 percent of diabetic patients who have foot amputations are smokers. It is rare for a nonsmoking diabetic person to lose a foot in this way.

The best method to reduce your risks is to stop smoking completely and immediately. Studies have shown that the damage to your lungs done by years of smoking can, in many cases, be repaired by your own body after you quit smoking.

There are many techniques available to help you stop smoking. Get your physician's advice on which method will suit you best.

After you give up the cigarette habit, make sure that you don't substitute an eating habit for it. Many ex-smokers tend to overeat during the first few months after they have kicked cigarettes. Overeating, as you know, will lead to being overweight, which may throw your diabetes management program into a tailspin. This is also a good time to start an exercise program since stopping smoking will increase your ability to exercise properly.

STRESS

One of the more difficult problems in diabetes management is stress and its many effects on your body. When you are faced with stress, your body responds with what is called a "fight-or-flight" pattern. Your body's systems pour out adrenalinelike substances to prepare your body for vigorous efforts in response to a stressful situation. At the same time, your adrenal glands release more cortisol, which inhibits insulin action and results in a rise in blood glucose. Physicians have found that persons in stress-producing jobs are more prone to develop type 2 (non-insulin-dependent) diabetes and are more difficult to treat when they do develop diabetes. In some persons, a condition called stress-induced diabetes occurs, which disappears when the stresses are removed.

How to handle stress is something everyone should learn, especially persons with diabetes. If you are measuring your own blood glucose, you can pinpoint what specific emotional stressors do to your glucose levels. You can then anticipate or correct any glucose increase with an appropriate dose of insulin.

Although you can't avoid all stress, you'll want to develop a plan to help you manage your response to stress. One way is to develop your own "mental health spa"—a little space and a little time set aside to help you relieve daily pressures. Imagery, yoga, and meditation are all helpful. Another way to handle stress is to exercise. The case for exercise as a means of reducing tension grows daily. Exercise challenges the spirit as well as the body and has a bonus effect for the diabetic person because it helps to lower blood glucose levels.

PILLS AND MORE PILLS

You will do yourself a big favor if you eliminate any unnecessary medications you may be taking. The sixteenth-century Swiss physician Paracelsus wisely noted that the only difference between a drug and a poison is the dosage. Americans tend to be a nation of pill poppers, seeking the magic potion to solve all ills. Persons with diabetes, in particular, should avoid unnecessary drugs as well as many of the health and nutrition fads that may actually worsen diabetes or its complications. When in doubt, check with your doctor.

One of the most worrisome medications for diabetic women is the birth control pill and its counterpart in later life: postmenopausal hormone replacement. Estrogen and progesterone affect the body's glucose tolerance. Insulin action may be inhibited in the presence of these hormones, and a woman who has a confirmed high blood glucose level should adjust her insulin dosage to keep the blood glucose levels normal. There are now "mini-pills" that avoid these problems. For postmenopausal women, a continuous steady dose of estrogen and progesterone will minimize any problems. Thus, there is no reason for a diabetic woman not to have the benefits of hormone replacement.

Water pills (diuretics) also pose problems for diabetic persons. In the past, they were often prescribed as weight reduction aids since they help to rid the body of excess water. However, diuretics have no effect on body fat and give a false sense of achievement regarding weight loss. They also interfere with diabetes control and actually lead to higher circulating glucose levels. Diuretics have proved helpful in treating persons with heart disease and/or high blood pressure, although in many cases, their use could be eliminated with appropriate weight loss and exercise programs. There are also better pills for treating high blood pressure.

HYPOGLYCEMIA

Since hypoglycemic symptoms may vary from one person to another, it is extremely important that you know its symptoms in *you*. With your glucose measurements, you will be in tune with your particular feelings when your blood glucose is too low. This is called hypoglycemic awareness training and is important for every person with diabetes. If you are in good glucose control, the first sign of hypoglycemia will often be a tingling in the mouth. You may not be able to read, watch TV, or even tell time well because your brain is the organ most sensitive to low glucose. Your skin may become cold and clammy and paler than usual. In addition, your breathing may become shallow and rapid and your eyes dilated. Some people develop headaches, trembling hands, and a tingling in the fingers, tongue, or other areas of the body. Still others describe buzzing in their ears, hunger, or tightness in the throat and tongue. The better your control, the gentler and more subtle the symptoms of hypoglycemia will be.

You may become somewhat clumsy during a hypoglycemic episode and have difficulty measuring your blood glucose. Your mood may also be affected and may range from feeling silly to uncontrolled crying, irritability, and unpleasantness with other people. Drowsiness, fatigue, abdominal pain, or sudden awakening from sleep may also indicate hypoglycemia. A common early symptom is hunger. A well-controlled, well-nourished diabetic person should not be unduly hungry unless hypoglycemic. But hunger may also be a sign of tension, anxiety, lack of sleep, or oncoming illness. In fact, about half of so-called insulin reactions or hypoglycemic episodes experienced by persons with diabetes may merely be hunger pangs provoked by other factors. Obviously not all these symptoms occur during hypoglycemia. One symptom alone may be the only indicator. The point is that you should be familiar with your particular set of symptoms and measure your blood glucose at the first sign. You should also encourage those close to you to be aware of clues they can use to help you head off hypoglycemia. You will be amazed (and sometimes annoyed) at how often those close to you are more sensitive to your low sugars than you may be.

Another sign of hypoglycemia is a rapid pulse rate in the absence of exercise. You have already determined what your resting pulse rate is as part of your exercise program. If you have a watch with a second-hand sweep, count your pulse for fifteen seconds and multiply the count by four to get your pulse rate. This is particularly useful when hypoglycemia symptoms appear and you have no means of measuring your blood glucose. There are several places where you can take your pulse: at the wrist, at the temple, or on the neck (see Figure 10.1). If your pulse rate exceeds what your highest resting pulse is *by even a fraction*, you should assume hypoglycemia (a blood glucose of less than 60 mg/dl) is occurring unless there are obvious precipitating factors such as anger, fear, or exertion. When in doubt, measure your blood glucose if at all possible. If not, take your *calibrated* sweets—the worst you will do is elevate your blood glucose level about 60 mg/dl.

If your blood glucose is less than 70–80 mg/dl, you should consume enough fast-acting sugar to raise it back to 100 mg/dl. For instance, if your blood glucose is 60 mg/dl and your calibrated sweets are each 20 mg/dl, you should take two pieces—no

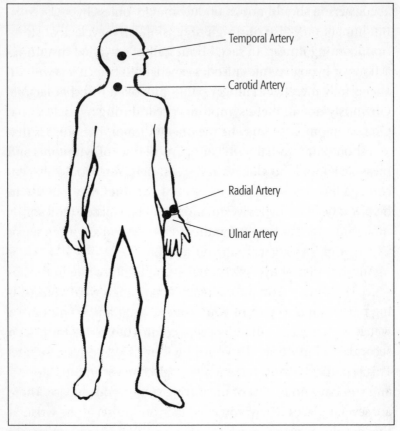

Temporal Artery

Carotid Artery

Radial Artery

Ulnar Artery

Figure 10.1 Pulse Points

more, no less. Wait twenty minutes. If the symptoms persist, measure your blood glucose again. If it is still less than 80 mg/dl, take another sweet. With practice, the repeated consumption of sweets will rarely be necessary.

Once you are in good control, it will become increasingly possible to prevent episodes of hypoglycemia. After a while, you will sense when your blood glucose goes below 80. If you measure a blood glucose below 70 mg/dl, drink a glass of milk, wait fifteen minutes, and repeat your blood glucose measurement. If you are still low, have another glass of milk and repeat your blood glucose in fifteen minutes. If you are still low, have a glass of milk and one slice of bread. This protocol has been especially helpful for children and pregnant diabetic women, and step three (milk and bread) is almost never necessary. Usually a glass of milk raises blood glucose 20 mg/dl and holds it there.

At first, the temptation to eat something before measuring your blood glucose will be overwhelming. You should resist, however, except when symptoms are so extreme that you no longer have the coordination needed to measure your glucose. In such instances, take only enough food to raise blood glucose about 60 mg/dl, and wait until your coordination returns. As soon as you are able, proceed to measure your blood glucose and take more carbohydrates only if indicated.

It is not uncommon for diabetic persons to treat hypoglycemia with sweets and then, without waiting for the subsequent rise in blood glucose, consume a mass of protein or a mixed protein-carbohydrate snack to satisfy their overwhelming hunger. The consequences of this approach are easy to predict: within two to three hours, most of the unplanned protein will appear in the blood as glucose. If the snack includes carbohydrates, the blood glucose may rise within an hour. Then the blood glucose roller coaster starts on its course, with high peaks and frightening lows. Instead, calibrated sweets or milk, followed by a ten- to twenty-minute wait before further eating will alleviate the ravaging hunger of hypoglycemia much more effectively than half a pound of cheese or a jar of peanut butter. You will also avoid a two-day catch-up period after "overdoing" it.

A diabetic person in good control with built-up glycogen in the liver and muscles should never experience the extreme situation of unconsciousness. But this may happen, and you should be prepared with a supply of glucagon, a hormone which counteracts insulin and mobilizes glucose in the bloodstream. It is injected just like insulin, and family or friends should be taught how to mix and administer it. Diabetic persons should include glucagon in their kit, with instructions for its use. As soon as consciousness returns, calibrated foods can be administered as usual.

As noted earlier, the injection of 15 "units" of glucagon from an insulin syringe will raise blood glucose about 30 mg/dl for three hours. This is very useful if you find your sugar dropping but are also sick and vomiting—as may occur, for example, during a bout of flu or morning sickness.

It is unlikely that this severe type of reaction will occur once good control and conditioning have been achieved. Good control results in a healthy liver with a ready supply of glycogen to counteract hypoglycemia. Therefore, the best way to avoid reactions is to be in good control and good physical condition. It is better to prevent hypoglycemia than to react to it.

LONELINESS, ANGER, AND FRUSTRATION

Lack of knowledge about diabetes and an inadequate management and support program frequently result in anger, frustration, and loneliness for the person with diabetes. Urine glucose tests and infrequent office blood glucose determinations will not provide enough information for you to take charge of your diabetes. Fortunately, modern technology and better management guidelines gives you the tools to monitor your own blood glucose and take control of your diabetes in any given situation.

The fact that you have this ability to help solve the many problems of diabetes will take away a good deal of the anger and frustration you have felt in the past. In addition, it will make you a partner with your physician and health care team in the management of your diabetes.

One of the best ways to learn more about diabetes and take away some of the loneliness associated with it is to talk to others who are in the same boat as you. Most communities have an American Diabetes Association, a Juvenile Diabetes Foundation chapter, or a Diabetes Club where you can meet other individuals who are also learning to live with diabetes. The internet now has several diabetes forums. CompuServe has one of the longest running and most useful groups. Learning together to adopt new and healthier lifestyles will make the task not only easier but also fun. These learning exchanges will be helpful to everyone and offer a basis for new friendships. Many diabetic persons get together in these groups to compare notes on a regular basis. (To locate the diabetes organization in your area, contact the national headquarters: American Diabetes Association, 1660 Duke Street, Alexandria, VA 22314; Juvenile Diabetes Foundation, 120 Wall Street, New York, NY 10005).

The best way we all learn is though role models, persons who are doing or have done what we would like to do and who can show us the way. You can read about such people in many books, pamphlets, and magazines published for persons with diabetes. The more you read, the more people you talk to, and the more you come to know your own responses through testing your own blood glucose, the better equipped you will be for any situation.

As you talk to someone else with diabetes, you will find that not only will your anger and frustration about the disease disappear, but you can take pride in the fact that you are doing well. In a sense, you are a member of a unique community of individuals whose condition has given them a special knowledge about living that is helpful to everyone. Because of your knowledge of nutrition, body metabolism, and responses to exercise and stress, you have a great deal to offer your nondiabetic friends. Once you realize this and put your knowledge to work for you,

you will acquire a sense of satisfaction in taking charge not only of your diabetes, but of your life itself.

INJECTING AND TESTING IN PUBLIC

Many persons with diabetes are reluctant to test their blood glucose or inject insulin in public. However, both tasks can be done without offending another person's sensibilities. Unlike urine testing, blood glucose analysis is socially acceptable. We live in a technological age, and people are fascinated by new gadgets. You will find that people not only are not offended by what you are doing, but are genuinely curious and eager to learn about it. Many may ask you to test their blood, too!

Diabetic persons are sometimes shy about injecting insulin in public because they feel this identifies them with drug addicts. Remember, this is a highly admired skill when done properly, and physicians were doing it long before addicts did. You can help others overcome their squeamishness about injections by explaining what you are doing and why. These explanations will gain you friends and will make it easier for them when they visit a physician. With the new pen devices or a pump, it is even easier to administer insulin without anyone even noticing.

Glossary

Acarbose A starch blocking glucose lowering agent.

Acetohexamide An oral hypoglycemic agent marketed under the brand name of Dymelor.

Acidosis A condition in which the amount of acid in the bloodstream increases. In diabetes, the most common forms are ketoacidosis, which occurs when a diabetic person has too little insulin and ketone bodies increase in the bloodstream, or lactic acidosis, which occurs when a diabetic person has excess lactic acid.

Adrenaline A substance (also called *epinephrine*) produced by the adrenal glands, which rest above the kidneys. Adrenaline can raise blood glucose levels and make a diabetic person more resistant to a given amount of insulin.

Alpha cell A type of cell in the pancreas gland that secretes glucagon.

Aneurysm A dilation or ballooning of the wall of a blood vessel.

Basal Insulin The insulin dose or secretion from the pancreas that controls glucose levels while not eating.

Beta cell A type of cell in the pancreas gland that secretes insulin.

Biguanide A type of oral drug (available as metformin).

Blood urea nitrogen A metabolic waste product found in the blood. It must be excreted through the kidney.

Bolus Insulin The insulin dose or secretion from the pancreas that covers the glucose absorbed from food.

Carbohydrate A fuel or energy-producing food for the body that can easily be changed into simple sugars, mainly glucose. It is the most readily available fuel for the body.

Cataract A clouding of the lens of the eye.

Chlorpropamide An oral drug (brand name, Diabinese) used to lower blood sugar.

Cholesterol A substance found in the bloodstream that may contribute to atherosclerosis (a disease of the large blood vessels).

Conjunctiva A thin membrane that lines the eyelids and covers the exposed surface of the eyeball.

Cornea A uniformly thick transparent membrane that protects the front of the eyeball.

Creatinine A substance that is a component of urine and a product of tissue breakdown. Creatinine accumulates in the bloodstream if the kidneys do not work correctly.

Diuretic An agent that increases or promotes urination.

Euglycemia A state in which the blood glucose level is in the normal range (50 mg/dl–150 mg/dl).

Exudate Fluidlike material that passes through the walls of vessels into adjacent tissues or spaces in inflammation.

Fat A fuel that is available for the body to use for energy, although not as rapidly as carbohydrates and proteins. Fat that is not used immediately is stored in fat cells until it is needed.

Fiber A part of plant material that resists digestion by humans.

Fibrinogen A protein in blood plasma that aids in the coagulation (clotting) of blood following an injury.

Glimepiride A sulfonylurea glucose lowering agent marketed under the brand name of Amaryl.

Glipizide A second-generation oral hypoglycemic drug (brand name, Glucotrol) now available as a generic drug. It comes in short and long acting forms.

Glomerulus A part of the kidney that filters blood to make urine.

Glucagon A protein hormone secreted by the alpha cell of the pancreas gland which raises blood sugar levels. Glucagon helps diabetic persons mobilize stored sugar and, as a result, counteract hypoglycemic reactions.

Glucose The most common simple sugar, also known as dextrose or blood sugar. It is the chief source of energy for humans and many other animals.

Glyburide A second-generation oral hypoglycemic drug (brand names include Diabaeta and Micronase). Now available as a generic and in long and short acting forms.

Glycogen The main storage molecule of glucose. Glycogen can be readily converted into glucose.

Glycosylation The process of linking glucose to another substance, e.g., hemoglobin.

Hemoglobin A protein found in red blood cells that carries oxygen to tissues throughout the body.

Hemoglobin A_{1c} A type of hemoglobin that has been modified by the addition of one or more glucose molecules. Once the glucose attaches to the hemoglobin, it does not come off. Measurement of hemoglobin A_{1c} is a useful way of finding out the average blood sugar over a period of three months.

Hyalin A clear substance that occurs in the breakdown of tissues. Its presence is a sign of kidney disease.

Hypercoagulable A term describing blood that tends to clot more readily than usual.

Hyperglycemia A condition in which the blood sugar is higher than normal.

Hypoglycemia A condition in which the blood sugar is lower than normal.

Insulin A protein hormone secreted by the beta cells of the pancreas gland. Lack of this hormone results in diabetes mellitus.

Iris The colored part of the eye between the cornea and the lens.

Islets of Langerhans A mass of small cells in the pancreas gland that contains alpha and beta cells. The beta cells secrete insulin and the alpha cells secrete glucagon.

Juvenile-onset diabetes mellitus A type of diabetes acquired during childhood or adolescence and requiring the injection of insulin for therapy. Also called insulin-dependent diabetes or type 1 diabetes.

Ketoacidosis *See* Acidosis.

Ketone bodies Highly acidic substances formed during the digestion of fat. They include acetone, acetoacetic acid, and beta-hydroxybutyric acid.

Lactic acidosis *See* Acidosis.

Laser A device that produces a beam of light of a specific wavelength that can be focused into a specific area. Lasers are being used to treat diabetic retinopathy.

Lens The transparent part of the eye just behind the iris. It focuses light rays to form an image on the retina.

Lipid Another word for dietary fat.

Lipodystrophy A scientific name for changes in fat tissue. Signs of this condition are little hollow places or bulges in the skin where insulin has been injected.

Lipoprotein A compound that contains both protein and lipid. Lipoproteins in the blood tend to carry cholesterol and be related to atherosclerosis. There are three kinds of lipoproteins. Very low density lipoproteins (VLDL) primarily carry triglycerides. Low-density lipoproteins (LDL) primarily carry cholesterol and deposit it in blood vessels. LDLs are considered a risk factor for atherosclerosis when present in relatively high amounts. High-density lipoprotein (HDL) primarily carry cholesterol, too, but they carry it away from the blood vessels. Therefore, they are thought to protect against atherosclerosis.

Lispro insulin A new "designer insulin" that peaks very rapidly and has a very short duration of action.

Maturity-onset diabetes mellitus A type of diabetes acquired after puberty and treated by meal planning alone or a combination of meal planning and oral hypoglycemic agents or meal planning and insulin. Also called non-insulin-dependent diabetes or type 2 diabetes.

Maturity-onset diabetes of youth (MODY) A rare type of diabetes, acquired during childhood or adolescence, in which the patient has significant circulating insulin levels. Persons with this form of the disease may not require insulin. Even though they developed diabetes when they were young, they tend to be more like persons with maturity-onset diabetes.

Metformin An insulin sensitizing drug that is useful for the treatment of type 2 diabetes.

Myopathy A disease that affects muscles.

Neuropathy A disease that affects nerves and their function.

Optic nerve A cablelike structure that carries visual impulses from the retina to the brain.

Oral hypoglycemic agent A medication that lowers blood glucose levels and is taken orally (by mouth).

Oxytocin A protein hormone that is made in the pituitary gland. It causes contractions of the uterus and can be used to stimulate uterine contractions that, in turn, can be monitored to make sure the baby is all right during pregnancy.

Pancreas A gland located in the back of the upper mid abdomen. It contains the beta cells, which produce insulin, and the alpha cells, which produce glucagon. These cells are found in the islets of Langerhans.

Photocoagulation A process that uses laser beams to repair damaged retinas.

Pituitary gland A gland that lies at the base of the skull. It produces a number of hormones which control other glands in the body.

Placenta An organ that exchanges substances between the fetus and the mother. It produces a number of hormones that help maintain both the fetus and mother during pregnancy.

Platelets Blood components that circulate in the bloodstream and contain no hemoglobin. They help form a blood clot to stop bleeding. Diabetic persons tend to have more active platelets and thus form clots more easily than do nondiabetic persons if glucose levels are high.

Protein A fuel for the body that is used more slowly than glucose. Protein is broken down into smaller particles called amino acids, the body's building blocks.

Repaglimide A drug that helps the pancreas secrete extra insulin.

Retina The delicate, multilayer portion of the eye that receives light and conveys images to the brain.

Retinopathy A condition in which the retina becomes injured or diseased.

Secondary complications of diabetes Problems associated with diabetes mellitus that are not related directly to acidosis or insulin deficiency. They tend to result from exposure to high glucose levels over months to many years.

Sugar A class of compounds that contain carbon, hydrogen, and oxygen. Simple sugars can combine to form complex sugars or starches or combine with other types of molecules, including lipids and proteins.

Sulfonylurea A class of drugs that are taken orally to lower blood sugar.

Tolazamide A sulfonylurea type drug marketed as Tolinase.

Tolbutamide A sulfonylurea type drug marketed as Orinase.

Triglyceride A type of fat or lipid circulating in the blood that is regarded as a risk factor for heart and blood vessel disease.

Troglitazone An insulin sensitizing drug.

Tubule A part of the kidney that collects and processes filtered urine from the glomerulus so that useful materials are reabsorbed into the body and waste products are excreted.

Type 1 diabetes The type of diabetes that results from an autoimmune attack on the insulin secreting cells of the pancreas. It was formerly called juvenile onset diabetes but, in fact, can occur at any age. The end result is a loss of insulin secretion and hence persons with this type of diabetes need insulin from some other source.

Type 2 diabetes The type of diabetes that results from insulin resistance. Because insulin continues to be secreted by the pancreas, oral agents can often be used for treatment. It used to be called adult onset diabetes. However, it can also occur in childhood.

Vitreous humor A clear, jellylike substance that supports the interior part of the eye between the lens and the retina.

Index